Stroke
Survivors

Stroke
Survivors

William H. Bergquist,
Rod McLean,
and
Barbara A. Kobylinski

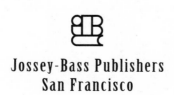

Jossey-Bass Publishers
San Francisco

Substantial discounts on bulk quantities of Jossey-Bass books are available to corporations, professional associations, and other organizations. For details and discount information, contact the special sales department at Jossey-Bass Inc., Publishers (415) 433-1740; Fax (800) 605-2665.

For sales outside the United States, please contact your local Simon & Schuster International Office.

Jossey-Bass Web address: http://www.josseybass.com

Library of Congress Cataloging-in-Publication Data

Bergquist, William H.
　　Stroke survivors / William H. Bergquist, Rod McLean, Barbara A. Kobylinski. — 1st ed.
　　　　p.　　cm. — (Jossey-Bass health series)　(Jossey-Bass social and behavioral science series)
　　Includes bibliographical references and index.
　　ISBN 1-55542-669-7
　　1. Cerebrovascular disease—Psychological aspects.　2. Cerebrovascular disease—Case studies.　I. McLean, Rod, date.　II. Kobylinski, Barbara A., date.　III. Title.　IV. Series. V. Series: Jossey-Bass social and behavioral science series.
　　RC388.5.B463　1994
　　616.8'1—dc20　　　　　　　　　　　　　　　　　　　　　　　　　　　　94-11647

The *Caregiver's Bill of Rights* in Chapter Fourteen is reprinted with the permission of Alzheimer's Society of Northern California.

"Ten Steps to Loving Yourself" in Chapter Fourteen is from *Ten Steps to Loving Yourself* by Louise Hay. Compton, Calif.: Hay House, 1993. Reprinted with permission.

HB Printing　　　　　　10　9　8　7　6　5　4　3　2

Contents

PART FOUR

Helping the Survivor

Preface

The percentage of stroke survivors has increased dramatically since 1950, making strokes a major cause of long-term physical disability in the United States. Extensive research has been done on the physiological and physical adjustment to strokes. This research has been effectively conveyed to stroke survivors through many excellent publications distributed by the American Heart Association or made available through other sources. But until recently, we knew little about psychological issues confronting stroke survivors.

We do know that depression, anxiety, and disruption of sexual function frequently go along with recovery from strokes. While a few studies provide us with a first glimpse into the processes of adaptation to a stroke, they do not adequately address the complex processes associated with the psychological adaptation to strokes. We do not have a comprehensive portrait of the recovery process or recommendations for stroke survivors, personal (family, relatives, friends) caregivers, or professional caregivers regarding this recovery process.

In this book, we report on a study we conducted and reflect on our own experiences as men and women who have had strokes or have provided psychological services to the survivors of strokes. We offer stroke survivors and their caregivers an opportunity to listen to the stories told by other survivors and caregivers about poststroke feelings and processes. These stories are filled with the depression and anxiety that have been identified in many previous studies. However, they also reveal optimism and even a sense of excitement about the new challenges and self-insights that emerged from the stroke experience.

What Is a Stroke?

Many people think of strokes as somehow related to heart attacks, but they are more accurately thought of as *brain attacks* (a term being used more and more frequently by professionals in the field). A stroke is the disruption in the blood supply to the brain, either from outside or from within the brain. When the blood supply is cut off to one part of the brain, it does not receive the oxygen it needs and the result is damage to the brain cells. The medical term for stroke is *cerebrovascular accident* (CVA).

Many medical workers are skilled in educating patients about the trauma and aftermath of strokes. We urge you to consult with these professionals. Our study in no way replaces the need for expert medical diagnosis or treatment. What we want to share with you are some of the experiences of having, coping with, and recovering (partially or totally) from a stroke. The people we interviewed tended first to define a stroke as an event that is big, scary, and confusing. It doesn't seem to have any clear source and often brings about major changes in physical and mental functioning as well as transformations in physical appearance.

A stroke influences not only one's body and mind, but also one's relationships with others and—even more important—one's sense of self. Recovery truly requires a "recreation" of one's self-image and feeling of self-worth. This is at least as difficult as regaining one's bodily and cognitive functions, such as walking, eating, or talking; it is made more difficult because of the need to "rewire" one's brain and body. Hopefully, this book provides assistance to stroke survivors and caregivers in this challenging recreative process.

The Research Project

Our study was conducted with seventy stroke survivors from northern and central California, specifically from the San Francisco Bay Area and the Sacramento area. A broadly representative sample was selected, with more than one-fourth of the people being interviewed coming from so-called minority populations. Our central California stroke survivors are similar in attitude and life-styles to survivors living in many Midwestern and Southern communities in the United States, while those from the San Francisco area are representative of men and women from urban centers as well as from affluent and middle-class commuter communities in the United States. One half of these interviews were conducted between 1990 and 1992 by doctoral students at the Professional School of Psychology and by two of the authors, William Bergquist and Rod McLean. A further set of thirty-five interviews were conducted with stroke survivors and caregivers during the fall of 1992 by students in a master's-level program at the same school.

The interview schedule used in this study was developed by the authors and the graduate students in San Francisco and Sacramento who were conducting the interviews. While the interview schedule was much too long for anyone conducting a one-hour interview with stroke survivors and caregivers, it served as a solid guideline for the interviewers when they were working with the open-ended interviewing processes of this project.

Organization of the Book

Stroke Survivors is divided into four parts, each consisting of three or four chapters. Many of the chapters are written by Rod McLean, who is a stroke survivor. He offers a detailed personal account of having and recovering from a stroke. We supplement his chapters with others that contain the stories and insights from the seventy stroke survivors we spoke with.

Part One focuses on the stroke experience itself, as well as describing precursors to the stroke and the survivors' early poststroke experiences (usually in the hospital). In Chapter One, Rod offers his personal experiences and insights regarding the stroke. Chapter Two follows up by providing a synthesis of the experiences that many other stroke survivors shared with us. It also touches on factors that may have precipitated their strokes. In Chapter Three, we pick up the thread of Rod's

narrative, focusing on his early hospital experiences. Chapter Four concludes this first section of the book with a synthesis of our interviews
regarding the survivors' initial confrontation with the reality of their
strokes.

Part Two deals with the immediate aftermath of the stroke. The
stories in this section primarily concern the early rehabilitation process,
usually in a rehabilitation center. In Chapter Five, Rod picks up where
he left off in Chapter Three, offering unique insight into the rehabilitation process. Chapter Six provides a complementary survey of the
rehabilitation experiences of the other stroke survivors we interviewed.
It also discusses perhaps the most important phenomenon associated
with the rehabilitation process: the experience of being a "new person"
following the stroke. The next two chapters shift our attention from
internal matters to external relationships. In Chapter Seven, Rod
describes changes in his relationships with other people following his
stroke. Chapter Eight contains a more general analysis—based primarily on the interviews we conducted with stroke survivors—of the impact of strokes on personal relationships.

Part Three examines stories concerned with returning to the "real
world" and discovering or inventing a life-style built on the new realities and new sense of self emerging from the stroke recovery process.
Our account of this phase in the recovery process begins in Chapter
Nine with Rod's description of returning home. Chapter Ten focuses
on the changing realities of the stroke survivors' lives and is based on
the interviews conducted by our research team. In this chapter, survivors speak of what they have lost and gained from the stroke experience. Insights from survivors also provide the focus of Chapter Eleven.
This chapter synthesizes the responses to the question we asked at the
end of every interview: what would the survivor like to say to other
survivors that might help them with their own recovery?

Part Four offers another perspective on stroke recovery. It looks
at this process from the viewpoint of the caregivers—both personal (relatives and friends) and professional. All four chapters in this final section underscore the need to extend understanding and support to the
caregivers, who play such a critical role in the recovery process. Chap-

ter Twelve focuses on how family caregivers assist survivors in this process. Chapter Thirteen looks at what the family caregivers consider to be the gains and losses and lessons learned from their experience. In Chapter Fourteen, Barbara Kobylinski describes her experiences in helping survivors and their families. In Chapter Fifteen, she offers her thoughts on the processes of healing and letting go as a professional caregiver. Readers who want to know more about a typical rehabilitation process may wish to read these last two chapters first.

An epilogue concludes the book, in which Rod shares with us the lessons he has learned from his own experience and the ways he has been able to put these lessons into practice. This book synthesizes the lessons learned from individuals who have had to cope with a stroke that either they or someone close to them has experienced. What do they have to say about the recovery process? What can be learned from the many stories we heard regarding the critical factors in promoting successful recovery from strokes? What are the implications of our findings for future stroke rehabilitation programs and policies? Given that we are at a crossroads with regard to health care in the United States and are engaged in a radical reconceptualization of disabilities and recovery processes, the insights reported here should be of considerable interest to those involved in new perspectives and new policies. The millions who confront the awesome challenge of stroke recovery and caregiving need, want, deserve, and demand our compassion—and even more important, our understanding and assistance.

Intended Audience

Our primary audience is made up of stroke survivors and their caregivers. In reading this book, they can develop an increased awareness of the capacities still present in survivors as well as the limitations imposed by a stroke. The book is also meant to foster greater understanding and appreciation of the attitudes, skills, and knowledge needed to effectively cope with this major life intrusion. And the very act of sharing stories can speed the recovery process.

Health care providers and other concerned members of the health care community are a second audience for the book. We offer a coherent developmental portrait of people who have successfully coped with strokes. Using this portrait as a model, these leaders and helpers can more effectively address the distinctive needs of survivors of strokes and their caregivers and can help empower them. Unfortunately, the stories that many stroke survivors and caregivers have offered us too often contain instances of insensitivity or even indifference on the part of professional caregivers. These frequently overworked professionals can be excused for their own distress and fatigue—which can lead to insensitivity and indifference—as they confront the complex changes now occurring in health care facilities throughout our society. There is no excuse, however, for the seeming failure of at least some professional caregivers to fully appreciate the distinctive needs and goals of stroke survivors. This book hopefully will help increase this understanding and appreciation among these professionals.

Acknowledgments

We wish to express our deep appreciation to the people who agreed to be interviewed for this study. Such a project could not have been conducted without the generous cooperation of many stroke survivors and caregivers, who volunteered to share their insights into the complex and challenging processes involved in "the reconstruction of self." While their names have been changed and their identities sufficiently protected to preserve their anonymity, we thank them for agreeing to expose their experiences, hopes, and fears to unknown interviewers.

While many of our informants indicated that the interview gave them a wonderful opportunity to talk with someone (often for the first time!) about their stroke experience, they were most interested in the value of their experience for others who are also recovering from strokes. Hopefully we have earned the trust of these thoughtful men and women and have produced a book that will be of use to stroke survivors and those who care for them.

We also wish to acknowledge the extraordinary talent and commitment of our student interviewers. We've recognized their contributions of time, effort, wisdom, and words to this study by listing them as case contributors at the end of the book. We thank all of them for their exceptional work. And on a more personal level, we would like to express our deep appreciation for the care and respect shown by our life partners, Kathleen O'Donnell, Joette Scoma, and Gerry Kobylinski. They have all provided guidance, encouragement, support, and some much-needed editing for this book. We are indebted as well to mentors in our past—whether they be a grandmother (Anna Briesch), parents (Herb and Carol McLean), or colleagues (Robert Shukraft and Carol Howard)—for their constant encouragement and inspiration. We also wish to note our gratitude to the many health care workers—physicians, rehabilitation specialists, nurses, counselors, and teachers (notably Elizabeth Piccard and Christy Baker of Florida State University)—who have cleared a path for us in acknowledging the role that psychological factors play in the processes of rehabilitation. Finally, we even want to thank those few men and women who have said no to us—who have attempted to place unnecessary limits on us in terms of our personal accomplishments and the scope of this research. They have inspired us to try harder to clarify our goals for this study and for our individual lives.

June 1994

William H. Bergquist
Gualala, California

Rod McLean
San Rafael, California

Barbara A. Kobylinski
Sacramento, California

Stroke
Survivors

PART ONE

Having a Stroke

1

What's Happening to Me?

I'm Rod McLean. I'm a stroke survivor. As a matter of fact, a neurologist described my stroke as a "spontaneous hemorrhage from an angioma or arteriovenous malformation in the left parietal area." In other words, a blood vessel in the left side of my brain had a weak point and burst. And it hurt! I was told later that I was within seconds or minutes of dying. But I guess I was as lucky as I could be, for it just happened that one of the best neurosurgeons in the region was right there when I was carried into the emergency room. He jumped into action to open my cranium and halted the rupture within moments.

The big one! It sure was. I think it was a Wednesday, late afternoon. Patty—a friend of mine—and I decided to walk four or five blocks to the fast-food restaurant. About halfway back, something started happening. It was really strange! I was invaded by an instant and massive headache. Everything started to become different—I didn't know what it was. I looked at my feet, but they didn't seem as though they were mine. I had to concentrate to make sure they would do what they were supposed to, because I noticed that I was having a harder and harder time walking.

At the same time, Patty became aware that something was going on. When she asked me questions, I heard and understood everything, but then I couldn't understand that I was forgetting whatever it was she had said. Not only that, her voice sounded like an echo. I had no reference point and quickly became afraid; I was scared of the unknown.

I noticed the sun was too bright and that I was seeing things surrealistically. My walking became wobbly, but Patty helped me get home.

Gary and Rolf, close friends and roommates, were out in the front yard; they saw something was wrong. In a way, I guess I was relieved to see my friends because it gave me a sense of security. They could see that I was afraid and that I appeared disoriented. They asked what was wrong and, to no avail, tried to figure out something to relieve the situation. Meanwhile, I was staggering and falling around. I struggled to answer their questions and pleaded for help and solutions. Looking at Patty, I tried to reach into my right front pocket to get some money to give her so she could go get me some aspirin. But somehow I couldn't find the right words to convey my needs.

I was trying to do all these simple things at the same time, and nothing was working right! My friends didn't know what to do. They carried me upstairs and laid me down on my bed, saying that I would be all right. They left! I was in pain. Everything was so hot; my entire body was drenched with sweat. I tried to sit up to take my shirt off over my head. I had no balance; every time I fought to sit up, I kept falling back down. The last time I hadn't been able to sit up was when I was a baby! Inside I was screaming, but on the outside I had somehow forgotten how to do that. Next, I tried again and again to take my shoes and socks off—that was practically impossible, too. I'd reach for the laces, but my fingers would totally miss them and I'd fall over sideways. Eventually, my friends came back and saw that I was in worse shape than a few minutes ago. They both stared at me in the realization of my anguish, glanced at each other, and agreed that they should take me to the hospital right away.

Lying on my side, I was starting to completely lose it; I was not really in control of anything. About all I could do was force myself to remain conscious—not really alert, but only distortedly aware that something was happening. Gary and Rolf carried me, limp, to the car and poured me in. Gary raced to the emergency room as Rolf held on to me. My body was still sweating and I was so hot that I had to hang my head out the window. It was odd. All the sounds—my friends' voices echoing and the outside sounds, such as the rush of traffic, cars honking, the wind, and everything else—angered me to the point of extreme hatred. I felt like lashing out to destroy and eliminate the grating noises that became an overwhelming irritation. My brain was throbbing, exploding with pain. Everything around me was aggravating the problem. I wanted it all to stop!

When we got to the hospital, they carried me into the Emergency Room and put me on a gurney. I was in tremendous pain. I was lying on the bed—out of control. I wanted out! As I internally screamed to escape, my brain continued to grasp for explanations or solutions. At the same time, I had no control of my body; my limbs and torso were writhing back and forth. My instinctual body was trying to get away from this unbelievable pain, too. But since the brain didn't have control, the body was just fighting it all. A nurse came in and looked at me rolling around, obviously in outrageous pain. She held up two fingers and asked me how many I saw. Remember, I was still in a pure rage. When she made that request, my wrath exploded and destroyed my image of her.

I noticed my vision was warped and distorted, and the colors were skyrocketing and forming different patterns; it was like the grand finale of a fireworks extravaganza, and it was all happening in my mind. When I blinked my eyes again and again, I discovered that what I saw was the same whether my eyes were open or closed. Either way, I was *not* seeing things as they were in reality. "Oh my God, I'm blind!" I thought.

Then, for some reason the writhing and internal chaos seemed to cease. I didn't hurt, feel, or hear anything anymore, though I was still scared. I realized that up to that moment, I had been totally exuding anger and hatred. While I was consumed with this hatred, I felt that if I were physically able, I would have flailed about and crushed anything in front of me.

My thought process shut down. My mind's eye rapidly flashed before me scenes from my entire life—from birth to the present. I was floating away into another dimension as if I were watching myself; maybe my spirit was separating from my body. In retrospect, it all seems so strange. Earlier, my body and mind had been working on instinct as I writhed and contorted, attempting to get rid of the horrendous anguish and all-encompassing pain. I had been fighting against death with ultimate fear. But all of a sudden, my entire being succumbed and then accepted what was happening. At that point, I felt I was floating in the "right" direction; I didn't resist anymore. The battle was over and I comfortably accepted my approaching death. I was exiting. I anticipated a new future in a new dimension. Then, I believe I was brought back to life by the brain surgeon. I was redirected into a deep sleep (or coma) and did not regain consciousness until twenty-one days later, when I awoke into the so-called reality of Tacoma General Hospital's Intensive Care Unit.

Let me explain a bit of what had happened. I had had what's commonly called an *aneurysm*, or ruptured blood vessel in the brain. The brain has many different sections, each with different functions in the overall "system." When the blood vessel exploded in the left hemisphere, a major "glitch" occurred in the communication area—the area that controls our abstract thinking processes as well as our physical movements, fine motor control, sense of balance, and other functions. My aneurysm caused the loss of at least three of the five senses: touch, hearing, and vision. I don't know if I lost smell or taste.

When my stroke happened, it was as if the system shut down. All of the physical components of my body transferred energy to where the emergency was. Unfortunately, this is the sequence that one's body follows, not only when it is reacting to a crisis, but also when it is about to die. I was told later that I had been in critical condition. My parents and friends were informed that I would be dead within ten to fifteen minutes if the brain surgeon didn't operate and snip the area of my brain where the bleeding occurred. The doctors anticipated that I would be confined to a wheelchair and unable to communicate for the rest of my life—a vegetable, a rutabaga. But I turned out to be an artichoke— "prickly on the outside, with a wonderful heart on the inside" (to quote an extraordinary man and advocate for the disabled, Ed Roberts)!

One thing that was so odd was that the brain attack happened when I was only twenty years old. (The stroke definitely sped up my maturation process!) At that time, I admittedly had no knowledge of what a stroke was; as a matter of fact, I didn't even know what a disability was. At that age, I had no conception of disabilities or fatal traumas—I still had a young adult mind-set and thought I was invincible. I was only beginning to mature.

To review my life briefly, I was raised by wonderful parents of mid-Canadian stock—Herb and Carol. They taught me by example and showed me how to love, care, share, and believe. They instilled in me the desire to never give up, and to search for and find the necessary miracle. I had four brothers and one sister, all younger. We lived in a suburb outside a medium-size city. I guess my upbringing was pretty conventional, with a backbone of strong principles.

At twenty, I was at least attempting to develop some maturity in regard to responsibilities. In retrospect, I see I was trying but resisting, too. I was having my second, terrible year of college; whatever the subject matter, I would have done better if I had attended or studied more. I wanted to do it all well, but at the time, I needed to explore my world and find out who I really was. I should have gone to Europe or somewhere else for a while just to get the itch out of my system; I needed some kind of experience so I could get a handle on myself and find a direction with fewer distractions. I continued college mainly because I wasn't sure which way to go. I was pulled toward travel and exploration, but I also felt obligated to follow a prescribed route, and I resisted that. I wanted to plot out a career plan but at the same time, I was attempting to get a full-time job to increase my cash flow. I was trying to get a reliable car to get around in as well. I was dabbling with the idea of trying to save some money to invest it or buy a house. In short, I was trying to build a life, but I was in conflict because I felt I hadn't experienced enough yet. So what did I do? I compromised and bought some time while I was in limbo. Another attempt to mature was in relation to my girlfriend: she and I dated a while, then became more serious and went steady. In our third year, we got engaged and "played house" while living in two separate homes. I was trying to develop something that I wasn't sure I wanted, but I was being pressed to make some decisions. I was really out of balance—I neither knew how to make a commitment nor wanted to. (I was a living example of the Peter Pan syndrome.)

My young life was full of all sorts of difficulties; new problems kept building up and I didn't know what to do with them. It was overwhelming! Problem after problem—each made it all worse. It seemed as if everything I touched exploded right in front of me. There was one hurdle after another. After one such dilemma, I was reviewing how devastating this year had been. I thought, "Boy, with all that I've been going through, nothing could possibly be worse." *Wrong!* A higher power threw a wide curve at me; either He was making a point with the stroke or He's got a weird sense of humor!

Right from the start, I want to address a key issue. Even though I had my stroke when I was comparatively young, I believe I share a powerful common ground with every "brain attack" survivor, regardless of age. We are all connected, in that we have confronted death. Also, because we were all derailed from our regular track and discovered that we had to begin anew, at the very least, we see things very differently from others.

I would appreciate it if during the course of your reading you would relate to the heart of these experiences rather than focusing on age. Yes, there are some differences in regard to age—stages of life, insights, levels of maturity, relationship to society, and so on. But when you have a brush with death, you become humble; you have seen or felt the "other side." You learn what's truly important and you start reprioritizing your new life. You relate to your survivor peers without age being a factor. There's a "badge" earned in surviving this major blow. Millions of us have been down the same path.

2

The Stroke Experience

In our adjustment to any major intrusive experience—whether it be illness, war, or personal failure or success—the stories associated with the beginning of the intrusion are critical, for they not only preserve the history of the experience and remind us repeatedly that it really occurred and affected us and others around us, but they also contain important themes and lessons to be learned about the nature and purpose of the intrusion. We try to find meaning in all of the major events in our lives, in hopes that we can learn something about how we should lead our lives in the future. That certainly is the case with regard to strokes.

In this book, people who have survived strokes speak about what happened to them at the time, about the responses (or nonresponses) of other people and institutions to their strokes, and about the immediate impact of the experience on their life. These stories help to guide the stroke survivors' own psychological adjustment to both the limitations and the new potentials presented by the stroke. They contain valuable insights about the survivors and their coping strategies. We must, therefore, listen closely to them.

In Chapter One, we read Rod McLean's story—about his vivid experience of surviving a massive intrusion in his life. What about the seventy stroke survivors that we interviewed? Are they like Rod? What are their stories about? What is it like to have a stroke? Is it painful? Is it frightening? What do these survivors choose to recount and highlight regarding their stroke experience? Are there many common themes in the stories told by these survivors, or does each seem to tell a different story? In this chapter, we first describe the distinctive experiences of eleven stroke survivors and identify several themes that seem to be present in each of their stories. We then make several more general statements about the experiences of these and other stroke survivors. The final section deals with the factors that may have caused their strokes.

Initial Stories

Carla's stroke occurred on an afternoon when she was waiting for her husband to come home to take her to a doctor's appointment. She was sitting at the kitchen table drinking some juice. She said the glass tipped over and she knew something was wrong. Carla knew she shouldn't remain sitting at the table but should get across the room to the couch. She crawled to the couch, got onto it, and sat waiting for her husband. She did not lose sight or consciousness. She noted that she did not feel pain or fear. She felt tired and uncomfortable, and she vomited. However, with all this, Carla reported having an I-don't-care kind of feeling.

When her husband came home, Carla told him she did not feel well. He canceled the doctor's appointment. He thought she was ill and disoriented from drinking, so he helped her get to bed. Later in the evening, he helped her to the bathroom and she kept falling off the toilet. That's when he realized there was something really wrong. He called for an ambulance.

Carla, like all stroke survivors, has undoubtedly often repeated this story—or probably would repeat this story if other people asked her about the stroke. What message does this story convey to other people (or to Carla herself, for that matter)? In her case, we apparently find the all-too-frequently reported story of "crying wolf one too many times." People who often complain unnecessarily about real or imagined ailments are not believed when they first experience the symptoms of a stroke. Alternatively, as with Carla or Rod, other family members or friends believe the stroke survivor is inebriated, drugged out, or simply tired after a long day of work or play. As a result, those around the stroke survivor often question the serious nature of their confusion and disorientation.

Margaret's stroke story began with a specific impact of the stroke, rather than with the stroke experience itself. She said that one of her nurses told her that she had almost died because she had gotten a piece of orange stuck in her throat when she had her stroke and no one knew it was there. Margaret went on to note: "I don't remember it, but I must have been eating an orange when I had the stroke. I remember a terrible pain in my head. It was the worst pain I ever had. It was behind my left eye." She added:

> I think it was my left eye but it could have been the right one. I don't remember anything again until some time the next day. There were bright lights that were awful and there was someone standing close saying, "[Margaret], can you hear me? Can you tell me where you are?" I don't know why I still remember that so clearly but I do. I didn't know why she was screaming at me. I couldn't answer and that was making me angry. "Oh yeah," they kept saying, "You don't have to be frightened . . . you are all right." Why do you think they kept saying "Oh yeah"? That made me angry too, isn't that strange?

Margaret's story seems to be about the frustration of losing control and the insensitivity of other people regarding this loss of control. We tell other people to "buck up" and not to be "afraid" when they have good reason to be depressed or afraid, especially early on during the stroke experience when they don't understand what's happening to them.

Bob's stroke happened in his sleep with no pain. He awoke and tried to go about his normal morning rituals of showering and shaving. He remembered "nothing worked" and experienced numbness and lack of coordination on his left side. Bob couldn't tie his shoes, buckle his belt, or get his body to do what he wanted. He felt panicky, though he guessed right away that he had had a stroke. He phoned his physician, who was also a personal friend, and the doctor tried to reassure him that maybe it was something temporary. Bob immediately feared that it was more serious and permanent. His wife drove him to the hospital, where he stayed for two days while a thorough assessment was made.

One of the themes in Bob's story appears to be that you can only trust yourself. Even a competent, trusted friend—who is also a physician—can be wrong. Bob's story is a clear statement about the importance of autonomy. But while such a story can be vindicating for a stroke survivor who was not believed, it can also lead to isolation and the inability of a survivor to accept appropriate assistance from family, friends, or members of the medical profession.

Jim's stroke came as a complete surprise. In fact, he was not aware that he had suffered a stroke. He had felt no pain and experienced no fear. Jim remembers driving back to his family's home after a day of skiing. He reports being very tired and deciding to go to bed at about 6:00 in the evening. It was not until Jim's girlfriend learned that he "had been drooling and dropped a cigarette on the rug" before he went to bed that she woke him and took him to the hospital. He was then examined, administered a brain scan, and told that he had suffered a stroke. Although he remembers very little of this incident, Jim maintains that he did not lose control, nor did he at any time lose consciousness.

The fact that Jim was not aware of the stroke and did not suffer any pain limited the physicians' ability to identify the actual location of the brain injury. Authorities later indicated that the stroke was caused by a vein in his neck "closing down." Jim's story offers a message that is opposite to that offered by Bob. Jim had people around him who cared about him and were knowledgeable. They got him to the hospital. This is a strong story about interdependence.

Beth had her stroke approximately two years before she was interviewed and was eager to tell her story. Prior to having the stroke, she was living alone. She described herself as a very social person, before and after the stroke, and enjoys visiting with friends and her adult children. She was tending her garden one day when she had a "funny feeling" on her left side and thought she was having a heart attack. Beth yelled to her neighbor for help. The neighbor came to her assistance, helping her into her house and then calling an ambulance.

Beth remembered feeling scared and talked about having many tests done in the hospital before she was brought to a room. She never lost consciousness. Her story seems to be a blend of both Bob's and Jim's, reaffirming both autonomy and interdependence. According to Beth, it's all right to be alone. However, it is only all right as long as you have a good neighbor.

Jane reported that she had a stroke at age sixty-two and that it was her first. On the day of her stroke, she was doing yoga on her living room floor. Her sister and husband were in the house, and it was raining. Jane said, "I suddenly felt something was wrong with me. My body felt different. I walked funny, like my legs couldn't hold me up. I went to an osteopathic doctor. He took my blood pressure and told me I was having a stroke. . . . I didn't believe him." Jane indicated that she "didn't know what a stroke was. I never knew anyone that had a stroke. . . . My husband took me to [the local hospital] and they didn't know if I was having a stroke, so it took them four hours before they admitted me." She was in the hospital for three weeks and recounted many disturbing experiences regarding the medical care she received.

Jane's story suggests the value of nontraditional expertise—in this case, osteopathic services—as opposed to traditional expertise (staff at the hospital). Like Rod and Bob, she advocates caution in depending on the expertise of other people. However, in her case caution is focused specifically on the medical establishment.

Grace indicated that she "woke up in the morning. I was very tired. I usually jump out of bed at 6:30." She got herself together for work, but she kept "feeling like I was going to tumble" and wanted to lie down. She felt something was "kind of wrong" but couldn't figure out what it was. She drove herself to work, although she continued to feel very tired. Getting out of the car, she kept dropping her purse. She went to the office but couldn't get the key in the lock. Her assistant came out and asked her what was wrong. Grace claimed "nothing," but he took her into the bathroom. Looking in the mirror, she saw that the "whole left side of my face was sagging."

Grace suffers from migraines and her assistant thought that was the problem, but she said she had already taken medication for the migraines. Two of her employees drove her to her husband's office. He brought her home and called the doctor, who told him to call an ambulance. Throughout this episode, Grace indicated that she wanted to maintain control, because she said "I'll be damned if I'll let them take me out on a stretcher." She lay down but fell off the bed because she couldn't control her legs. By the time the ambulance came, she was unable to stand up or walk and "was happy to go on the stretcher."

At that moment, Grace began the process of psychological adaptation to her stroke. She began to acknowledge her loss and allowed herself to be carried by others. She was in the hospital for about three weeks and then in a local rehabilitation center for about six weeks. For her, it seems to be important to allow other people to be helpful—the sign of a good manager. There is an important message in this story indicating that one doesn't have to control everything. Unlike with Bob and (to some extent) Jane, you can trust the expertise and intentions of other people.

Thelma remembers feeling fatigued and dizzy on a Thursday evening and lying down in bed. Her husband became alarmed when he noticed that her mouth looked "twisted" and called the doctor. She was taken to a nearby community hospital for observation, and the doctor told her then that he suspected that she had just had a "minor stroke." When she awoke the following morning, Thelma discovered that she was completely paralyzed. She reported that she felt no pain and that she immediately understood what had happened to her. She probably understood her condition because she is an experienced nurse. She was immediately taken to the intensive care unit, where she stayed for three days.

Thelma went on to note that her immediate reaction was one of terror, shock, and a sense of devastation. She said, "You go crazy when something like that happens." Within a few days of the stroke, she began to think of ways to get to a nearby bridge so that she could throw herself off. In her story, she certainly seemed to be describing a message of fear and despair. Even as an experienced nurse, she was unable to ward off the devastating impact that a stroke can have on one's sense of vulnerability and self-sufficiency. She knew what to expect. Perhaps that is part of the reason she was depressed. She knew what she'd be confronting in the future and knew it would be a difficult recovery process.

John experienced his stroke while he was asleep. He felt fine during the evening prior to the stroke and anticipated taking care of some work for his local Rotary Club the following morning. When he awoke in the morning, he was lying on the floor in a room he seldom used. His initial reaction was of surprise that he would even be in that part of the house. Once he realized that he could not move or speak, he became terrified. John remained on the floor for nearly an hour, anticipating that he would be dying at any moment. He recalls feeling at peace waiting for his mortal life to end and passed the time by praying and reflecting on his life.

After a while, he realized that he was not going to die immediately and that he should make an effort to get some help. He found it difficult to move at all but did manage to pull himself over to a wall he shared with his neighbor. He began banging on the wall, hoping to attract attention. Unfortunately, it was nearly an hour before he received help and was taken to the hospital. John offered us a story of religious faith — and also of self-reliance and perseverance.

Roberta experienced her stroke when she was driving to work with a friend. She said that she noticed some sensitivity in her right eye but that she did not become alarmed. She felt at that time that her contact lens was causing her some problems. She continued to drive but had to pull over when she lost sight in her right eye. She tried to tell her friend what was happening but had difficulty speaking — much as Rod was unable to communicate with his friends. Her friend decided to drive her home and call her personal physician. By the time they got to her home, Roberta was unable to speak at all and could not tell her friend her physician's name. She said that she was not scared but became increasingly frustrated because she could not verbalize what she wanted to say.

She then tried to write down her physician's name but found that she couldn't write his name even though in her mind she knew the correct spelling. Finally, she was able to find her physician's name in her address book and showed it to her friend. The friend called the physician, who arranged for an ambulance to take her to the hospital. Roberta said that she did not remember the ride to the hospital. The theme of creative problem solving seemed to pervade her story. She showed that she was capable of being creative, though her story also suggested that she failed to heed some telltale signs of a stroke.

Sheila was forty-eight years old and enjoying a day of swimming with friends at a lake when she suddenly became weak and had difficulty with her speech. In an attempt to walk toward the shore, she discovered that her body would not respond, and she had to be assisted from the water. Her friends were concerned but thought that the combination of alcohol and overexertion had caused her reaction. Sheila insisted she would be all right with some rest. However, when it appeared that her condition was becoming worse, a friend who happened to be a nurse was able to persuade her other friends to take her to the nearest hospital. A short while after the onset of noticeable symptoms, Sheila—under protest—was taken to a small seaside hospital some thirty miles away. She was not cognizant at that moment that this was a turning point for herself and her family.

Once at the hospital, the doctors and nurses seemed baffled about her condition. One of her friends (not among those swimming with her) reported arriving at the hospital about six hours after Sheila's admission. Sheila was stretched out on a gurney, exposed for all who wished to see. She appeared to be in a state of bewilderment. Her eyes kept darting around the room and her words were slurred. No physician was available at that time, and the nurses had arrived at the conclusion that nothing should be done until the alcohol wore off. Sheila's children, husband, and friends were waiting in confusion and apprehension.

Sheila remained in the hospital while her condition continued to deteriorate. Still, no diagnosis was given, no testing was done, and no treatment was administered. Usually, according to the friend (a trained nurse) who was reporting on the case, physicians would take CAT scans and ultrasound recordings and perform other procedures to determine whether the stroke was caused by bleeding or its opposite, a clot. Four days after her admission, Sheila's family consulted with their private physician and an emergency helicopter transfer was made to a hospital that could provide better treatment. Sheila underwent surgery immediately, and the family was informed that she had a 25 percent chance of becoming worse, a 70 percent chance of remaining in the same condition (no speech and paralysis on her right side), and a 5 percent chance of improving. Her future appeared bleak.

Sheila had suffered a stroke, devastating for both the victim and those closest to her. Her stroke was not typical. It apparently was brought about by an accident that occurred while she was diving into the water. The impact of her dive apparently severed a carotid artery in her neck—which, in turn, caused a blood clot to form in the left hemisphere of her brain. Sheila's early symptoms were not noticed because of the effects of the alcohol in her system. However, her oldest son stated that a glass fell from her hand shortly after the dive. It wasn't until a few hours after the accident that Sheila exhibited pronounced motor and speech difficulties.

Like many stroke survivors, Sheila offered a story that combined a component of personal fault with a component of other people's failure. Sheila's friends might have been quicker to discover her stroke if she had not been consuming alcohol. And, as in Jim's story, the hospital staff were to be faulted. Sheila's story also resembles that of many other stroke survivors in that it blends the themes of autonomy and interdependence. On the one hand, it conveys a sense that she (like Jim) is alone in the world and can't rely on other people (especially the so-called "experts"). On the other hand, her story conveys a sense (like Grace's story) that other people in her life will always be there for her—with their care and their expertise (specifically, her nurse friend).

General Findings

The features of the stories we've just touched on also tend to be reflected in the stroke experiences of the others we interviewed. First, the stroke experience itself seems to have either been very painful or not painful at all. Whether or not it was painful, the stroke inevitably was experienced as very frightening. For those who had little or no pain, the stroke was often even more frightening than it was for those with considerable pain, for the stroke came as a surprise—when they tried to get out of bed in the morning or when they tried to stand up after sitting in a chair. The level of fear and confusion seemed to be unrelated to knowledge about strokes, though Thelma may have become depressed in part because she foresaw the long recovery process that she would soon have to confront. People with considerable experience in the health professions, or who had previously dealt with their own strokes or strokes experienced by others in their family, found the stroke to be just as disconcerting as those who were naive about strokes and had no experience with other stroke survivors.

Why was the stroke so frightening? The loss of physical control certainly is a central feature. Georgia spoke of feeling "so, so helpless." Greta—a knowledgeable member of the health care profession and a stroke survivor—stated that she felt she would rather have had cancer than a stroke, because of the degree of disability and loss of independence associated with the stroke. She became quite depressed after having had her stroke. Many stroke survivors experience the loss of control primarily as a loss of physical control over their bodily functions. Many feel embarrassment along with frustration about this loss of control. Celeste lost control of her bladder and bowels when she had her stroke, which made her feel horrible.

Sean described his stroke as being overwhelmingly frightening because of his loss of control: "I was in terror. I was so afraid I would never regain the functioning I had lost. It was overwhelming." The professional who interviewed Sean noted that an intelligent, educated man like Sean had never known such a separation between his will and his body. The inability to control speech and thought for Sean was probably as profoundly embarrassing for him as was the loss of bladder control for Celeste. In both cases, they could compare the way they used to function with the way they now must interact with the world.

Another important element is the totality of the experience. Sheila described the shock of discovering that "the right side of my body was dead!" Georgia doesn't remember what happened to her, other than falling to the ground. "When I woke up," she recalled, "I felt bewildered, frightened, and shocked. I couldn't speak or move my left arm and leg. I started crying. I became hysterical. I didn't understand what had happened to me. I felt as if I had somehow died. It was a horrifying experience." Typically, when one has had a stroke, everything seems to go wrong at the same time. As Rod so vividly described, a stroke survivor typically can no longer walk, hold things, or even talk. With each attempt to do anything, we're reminded of our limits. For many stroke survivors, the most disconcerting experiences are associated with the loss of speech. Georgia observed: "I couldn't speak what I was thinking. It seemed like nobody could understand me. It was a nightmare."

Headaches, loss of vision, bright or flashing lights, and loud ringing in the ears often accompany physical incapacity. People are thrown onto what Georgia described as an emotional "roller-coaster." She said that immediately after she had her stroke, "I felt so frustrated, I wanted to die. I had no control of my body. I couldn't speak, so I didn't do anything. For a while, I felt like a vegetable. I felt like a little child. I didn't know who this person was that I became overnight. I felt 'dead' inside. And actually some part of me did die." Strokes often seem to throw people back to their infancy: they can't walk, talk, or even think clearly. Rod described the experience of looking in a mirror and seeing himself as an "adult baby." Survivors are suddenly absolutely dependent on the assistance of others, even if they don't lose consciousness.

As we will see throughout this book, personal and professional caregivers (including medical personnel) can play a helpful or a hindering role in the recovery process. If they treat survivors like children or are otherwise belittling, as apparently was the case with Celeste's doctors and nurses, the feelings of dependency and accompanying feelings of anger and depression can be exacerbated. The overall recovery process will probably also be impeded. But as we have tried to show, the survivors' own descriptions of the stroke experience can often provide valuable insights into the nature of the support they want and need from those who care deeply about a successful recovery.

Events Leading up to the Stroke

Rod had a number of hints that he was going to have a stroke during the year preceding his stroke. Furthermore, he faced many challenges during that year that proved to be psychologically and physically stressful—and that perhaps made him more vulnerable to having a stroke. Stress is one potential cause of strokes. Many physicians, medical researchers, and psychologists speak about the impact of long-term stress and even short-term intensive stress on physical well-being. Often, as Holmes and Rahe pointed out many years ago, the stress that helped to bring about a stroke or other physical ailment did not occur immediately before the stroke but may have occurred eight to ten months earlier (see Rahe, McKean, and Arthur, 1967; Holmes and Rahe, 1967).

We all have our opinions about what causes strokes, and frequently our perspective is tainted by our own biases regarding "wrong" or "bad" behavior. Strokes are caused by: too much liquor, too much hard living, too few vitamins, poor exercise, excessive sex, too much work, not enough work, too much aggression, not enough assertiveness, and so forth. Zelman (1992, p. 1) observes that the Hispanic survivors she knows tend to attribute strokes to *curage* (excessive anger), while "a Hmong family [said] that strokes are caused by negative spirits. An Afghani family expressed its concern [that] their mother's stroke was caused by 'too many worries on the brain.' Mainstream America has its own folklore for the cause of stroke—we use the term 'stress.'" Each of these theories about the major causes of strokes holds an important truth. In interviewing survivors regarding their stroke experiences, we asked about the events that occurred within a year before their stroke. They told us about three different kinds of contributing factors: (1) social relationships (and, in particular, family relationships), (2) health prior to the stroke (including knowledge about strokes and related health issues), and (3) personal and work-related issues. Following are some of the stories they offered regarding the factors that may, in our American folklore, have led to "stress" and, in turn, to the stroke.

Social Relationships

Most of the people we interviewed were married and many had children—though often the children were grown and no longer living at home. There were many gratifying examples of warm and supportive relationships with husbands, wives, and children—particularly when it came to their assistance after their loved one had a stroke. For example, Jane experienced substantial support from her husband before and after her stroke—both of these hard-working adults having retired less than three months earlier. Jane led an extremely active life before and after the stroke, finding herself with a large, extended family and many friends. Her support system during her recovery was remarkable—including the stroke support group that she attends regularly. Yet, even for Jane, there were problems associated with her significant relationships prior to the stroke. Her husband's retirement had brought additional stress to her life: "It was hard to be around him all the time. I do things real fast and I know what I want. He's really slow and that gets on my nerves."

Many of the stroke survivors spoke (often hesitantly) of problems in their marriage or in their relationships with their children. Susan's prestroke story exemplifies the fairly common problem of a marriage turned sour. During her twenty-five-year marriage, she had experienced verbal and physical abuse from her husband. He was very demanding, and as she stated, "He wanted me to wait on him as if I were a servant, [and] I thought that I was being a good wife by meeting his demands." In retrospect, "I was his slave." Susan's husband also refused to work: "All he wanted to do was fish." He was a "spoiled brat."

Like many women of her era. Susan was faced with a very demanding and almost childlike husband. She worked diligently to meet his needs (and those of her children). Although she was in a dysfunctional relationship, she continued to imitate her mother's model of a "good" housewife: self-sacrificing and noncomplaining. She was expected to work full time, take primary care of the children, and meet all of her husband's needs. He refused to work after being laid off in his fifties and was physically abusive in his relationships with Susan and the children.

Though not married, Mary—like Susan—spoke of an abusive relationship in her life at the time she had her stroke. She lived with a male friend who exploited her financially and physically abused her. Her environment was infused with alcohol and drug abuse. Such an environment cannot help but induce psychological and physical stress, which may culminate in a stroke or other illness. But Mary had failed to recognize that she was at risk until she had the stroke.

Other stroke survivors spoke about their sense of isolation from significant people in their lives. Often, these individuals had recently left their job (and close friends) because of retirement, had gotten divorced, or had seen their children leave the nest. Roberta is among those who live alone. She reported that she had met a noncommissioned officer (NCO) when she was in the army and stationed at an army base on the East Coast. They were married, but she said it was an unhappy marriage. She felt that some of their difficulties may have been related to her being an officer and his being an NCO. She stated that at that time, officers were strongly admonished not to fraternize with enlisted personnel, and here she was—a female officer married to an enlisted man. They got divorced in 1962; the divorce was bitter, and she has not had any contact with her ex-husband since then. They did not have any children. Roberta has never remarried or entered into any other commitments, either short-term or long-term. The only family she had at the time of her stroke were her pet cats.

Jim similarly was divorced when he had his stroke, having also served in the military (Air Force) as a captain. He was married for fourteen years during his military career. After his retirement, he was soon divorced; however, one of his two children from that union now lives with him. For Jim and Roberta, living alone may be a preferred way of life; however, after they had their stroke, this way of life no longer was viable. Jim's daughter has lent a hand. Roberta, however, is not as fortunate. She has no children and must rely instead on the support of friends.

Health Prior to the Stroke

Most of the people we interviewed reported good prestroke health. They usually were surprised by the stroke and knew of no physical warnings beforehand. Mary, for instance, was sixty-six years old and living at a board-and-care facility when she had her stroke. She reported that her health had been good and that other than a few problems with her teeth, she had no medical problems. Roberta was fifty-four years old when she had her stroke and was in relatively good health, though as we noted above, she felt isolated. John similarly reported that his health was relatively good at the time of the stroke. He admitted that he had slowed down but attributed this to his age and not to any medical ailments.

Georgia was a vital seventy-two-year-old Hispanic woman; she lived in New Mexico when she had her stroke: "It happened on New Year's Eve 1987. I was living with my oldest daughter and her husband then and am still living with them. . . . My health prior to my stroke was excellent. In fact, back in November of 1987, I had a complete physical done and I passed it with flying colors. I was feeling pretty good prior to the stroke."

While many of the survivors we interviewed created this overall rosy picture of physical health, this picture often changed when our conversations with them pushed back their examination of physical health a few months or even several years. There often were signs of physical illness—frequently associated with specific stressors. The stroke survivors tended to ignore or misinterpret these signs. Carla, for example, was fifty-four years old when she had her stroke. Previously, she was diagnosed with high blood pressure, and for many years, she had suffered from headaches. However, she reported that she "had no other warnings—the stroke occurred unexpectedly." Susan also reported that prior to her stroke she had experienced severe medical problems, notably multiple bouts of pneumonia, which the doctors later found to be related to heart disease. She had also experienced four or five ministrokes. Yet she never took these symptoms seriously and was surprised when she had a major stroke.

Similarly, Bob reported various signs of stress and physical illness. He now believes that he was "burned out" on his job before having a stroke. Furthermore, in retrospect he realizes that he was probably predisposed to strokes. His mother died of an aneurysm and his father died of a heart condition, in both cases when they were in their early sixties. He also reflects back on his own childhood and realizes that his Wyoming diet included a lot of beef and pork. He remembers his mother always telling him to "eat the fat, it's good for you." He now looks at his youthful life-style with disdain but recognizes "no one knew about cholesterol in those days." Yet, when he became an adult—and did know about diets and cholesterol—he failed to heed the warnings in his physical and psychological self that cautioned him to slow down and take better care of himself. Bob now knows better but didn't acknowledge his predicament at an early enough stage to avoid a stroke.

Sean was a fifty-one-year-old business executive when he had a stroke in 1991. He was in the middle of a career transition and was working intensively on a project in Canada. He traveled extensively but felt he was doing his best to manage his health adequately. Diagnosed with diabetes six years before, Sean was not able to regulate his diet while relying on restaurant food. He had been using insulin and attempted to take walks in the cities he was visiting in Canada. However, 1991 was a particularly busy year for him, and he did not keep close control of his diabetes. As was the case with many high-pressured businesspeople we interviewed, Sean had his stroke just when he finally decided to slow down and take a vacation. Sean, like Bob, knew at some level that things weren't quite right with regard to his physical self; yet it took a stroke to get his attention and shift his pattern of work.

Another of the stroke survivors we interviewed, Greta, had been a pharmacist for many years and grew up with a strong medical background. She indicated that she overlooked or ignored a variety of warning signals. The evening before her cerebral hemorrhage, she experienced an intense headache, which felt like a "tourniquet" around the back of her head. She took some painkillers and went to sleep. On awakening, she experienced no pain, but when she attempted to get out of bed, she was unable to make her body perform properly. She was paralyzed on her left side and actually took several steps before she realized what was wrong. The experience was very confusing for her (even though she is in a medical field), and it took a few moments before she understood that she had had a stroke. She managed to contact a neighbor, who called an ambulance to take her to the hospital.

Greta (like Carla, Bob, and Sean) should have heeded the warning signs. They all knew about strokes and about their deteriorating physical condition. Yet, in their own way, all of them tried to deny the implications of these symptoms. We will show throughout this book that at certain times during the stroke recovery process, the defensive strategy called *denial* can be effective and may, in fact, be essential to this recovery. Prior to the stroke, however, denial is inevitably counterproductive and often leads to serious physical trouble.

In other instances, the stroke survivors were simply unaware of what was happening to them. Many of the people we interviewed knew nothing about strokes and didn't have sufficient medical knowledge to connect any of their physical ailments to the impending stroke. Mary, John, and Georgia, for example, may have not been in the great state of health that they described when interviewed. They may have had several small problems that simply were not of sufficient magnitude to arouse their anxiety or even their attention. They remained unaware that the stage was being set for their stroke.

Like these three survivors, Jane indicated that prior to the stroke, her health status was excellent. However, she also reported that she had not been to a doctor for twenty-two years, so it's unclear whether she was fully informed of her health status. Her unexamined health is particularly serious, given that she had experienced substantial stress in her life prior to this stroke, as we noted above with regard to her highly demanding, retired husband. Similarly, for Alice, the physical conditions leading up to her stroke remain unknown and elusive. She can't really remember how she felt prior to the stroke—though she thinks that she was probably in pretty good health (having had a physical exam a short time before). Even after her stroke, Alice still doesn't quite know what happened to her or how she might avoid future strokes. Like Mary, John, and Georgia, Alice should be better informed about what a stroke is and how it is caused. Yet one or more of these survivors may have purposely ignored information they had been given, or they may have been unable to register or comprehend this information because of the cortical damage done by the stroke. Clearly, providing useful and understandable information about strokes and stroke prevention to the stroke survivors—and their caregivers—is a major challenge.

Personal and Work-Related Issues

Sheila was forty-four years old when many events affected her life and led, perhaps, to her stroke. She enjoyed excellent health until she had a ski accident that laid her up for several months. At about the same time, she separated from her husband of eighteen years and began making plans for a divorce. These changes were compounded by a shift in her parental status. She became a grandmother (with three other grandchildren on the way) and was once again in the role of mother (part time) to young children. She had also decided to move to a mountain resort and set up a new life independent of her ex-husband. The stroke followed soon after this move.

Thelma was initially unable to remember any unusual stresses during the year preceding her stroke but then recalled that she had been having trouble with her oldest daughter that year. The daughter had become homeless and delusional. Her son had a breakdown in high school— apparently a psychotic episode—and had subsequently been diagnosed as schizophrenic. Thelma was constantly worrying about the health and safety of both children. While her son has since received excellent treatment and her daughter is now living in her own apartment, Thelma's anxieties during this critical period may have contributed to her stroke.

Tom similarly experienced major problems with his son prior to his stroke. At the time of the stroke, he was visiting his son at a local hospital. Many things changed for Tom the night of the stroke. He describes being extremely concerned about his son, due to his extensive injuries. A tragic car accident had resulted in the death of two people and had left the son in a coma for three months, with a broken neck and back as well as a possible brain injury. While it was fortunate for Tom that he had his stroke while visiting the hospital, the stress associated with his son's massive injuries certainly added to whatever stress was already present in his life. His son's slow recovery since Tom's stroke has made adaptation to the stroke much more difficult—as is the case with other stroke survivors, like Thelma and Tom, who have had to confront other family-related problems along with recovery from their own intrusive life event.

Many of the others we interviewed were enmeshed in hectic life-styles when the stroke hit. Typically, these stressful experiences are of the type in which solutions and options are not readily available. Personal tragedies were often compounded by high levels of stress on the job. Jim experienced unusual stress at work, moved to a new home, and had to confront the death of his father—all within the year preceding his stroke. Roberta was employed as a civilian at a large army base when she had her stroke. She indicated during her interview that the job had become increasingly stressful and that this stress probably contributed to her high blood pressure. Like Jim, Roberta had experienced the added stress of a parent's death—in this case, her mother's—a year earlier. This stress was compounded when her mother revealed, just before her death, that Roberta had been sexually molested as a child.

Todd was similarly concerned about the stressful life he led prior to the stroke. His interviewer was struck during the interview with the "addictive quality" associated with events leading up to Todd's stroke. Todd spoke of many competing work and family obligations that had kept him very busy for at least the last thirty years prior to his stroke. He didn't know what to do with himself when he wasn't busy being a teacher, sculptor, and father to three children. These activities, according to Todd, kept him occupied every day from early morning through periodic late-evening work in the studio.

He also mentioned that one daughter and one son were adolescents living at home at the time of the stroke and said that this was a particularly stressful time for his family. Stress doesn't just come from negative experiences. Todd undoubtedly found much that was enjoyable in his work as a teacher and musician. His children, no doubt, were sources of great joy. These generally positive activities can still be stressful, however, and can have a negative impact on one's physical health.

Like Todd, Georgia spoke of leading an active life prior to her stroke and described it in a positive manner: "I had a wonderful year prior to my stroke. Things in my life were going pretty good. I always kept busy. I was involved with [a local church group]. We would travel all over the country. We would go play bingo, have dinners and dances. . . . Thinking back, I had a very good and happy year before this happened to me." The central question to ask in trying to discern the preconditions for Georgia's stroke is whether this level of activity and the associated stress were detrimental to her health.

For many adults, too little activity can be much more stressful than too much activity. The key factor is probably not the level of activity and stress, but rather abrupt (and often unwanted and unanticipated) changes in the level of activity. If I am accustomed to being active and heavily committed, then forced inactivity (as a result, for instance, of physical illness, retirement, or children leaving home) may be painful. On the other hand, if I am used to living a quiet and predictable life, then rapid change and the need for readjustments and high levels of activity may be stressful.

Perhaps for Georgia—who "always kept busy"—involvement in a church group was positive and contributed not to her stroke but to her successful recovery from this affliction. In her younger days, Georgia owned two convenience stores in New Mexico, which provided the focus of her life. She indicated that she worked long hours at both stores—about seventy-two to ninety hours per week—and that this didn't bother her at all. Continuing activity after she retired may have been critical. Forced inactivity may have been particularly difficult.

What about Todd? Was he accustomed to high levels of activity? Would slowing down have been even more difficult and stressful? And what about the loss of a social support system if Todd had dropped out of many of the activities in which he was involved? In our discussion of social relationships, we mentioned that several of the people we interviewed—like Georgia—had strokes soon after retiring from a long-term job. Retirement usually means the breaking off of important relationships. This is particularly the case if the retiree has devoted much of his or her energy and time to the job. In many cases, fellow workers are the only important relationships that the retiree has in life—other than family (and in some cases, family members aren't even around). Georgia was fortunate in that she was active in her church as well as her business ventures. Thus, she did not experience the frequent drop-off in personal contacts after retirement and was able to look to other members of the church for support after she had her stroke.

Retirement is stressful, however, for yet another reason. Many men (and some women) have defined their sense of self primarily in terms of their job. When they retire, they no longer feel important, nor are they appreciated by other people around them. They have been "put out to pasture" and no longer have much to contribute to the world. Eldon received a lucrative offer for early retirement from the gas company, having worked for the company forty-two years. He even became a consultant for the utility company on a part-time basis for six years after retirement. Yet he greatly missed the formal position of authority as well as the camaraderie. He had two strokes that he relates directly to his early-retirement decision.

Jane similarly indicated in her interview that she had "loved her job" and hated to leave it through retirement. Retirement is also difficult because retirees are no longer wage earners. Even with a substantial pension and social security payments, many people feel financially vulnerable, because they are no longer receiving regular paychecks. They must rely on retirement plans over which they have little control.

The relationship between stress and the occurrence of strokes and other physical ailments is related not just to accustomed levels of activity and challenge, but also to attitudes. How do we feel about the stress we are facing? Have we brought about the negative conditions ourselves, or do we feel powerless to influence the level and type of stress we are exposed to? Are we willing to live with the stress because we are moving toward some goal that is important to us, or are we simply pawns in a life game being played by forces that are much greater than us and that are seemingly indifferent to our welfare?

What about the stroke itself? Is it only a curse, or is it somehow defined as a hidden blessing? If it is only a curse—another problem forced on us by an uncaring world—it will become yet another source of stress and will lead to further physical dysfunction. What happens when stroke survivors take a more positive attitude? Bob was in his early fifties when he had a stroke. He's convinced that the stroke was related to the pace and pressure at which he was working—an appraisal very similar to those made by others. However, Bob saw the stroke as a blessing rather than a curse. He felt it was his body's way of slowing him down. While that is a heck of a way to get this message, he believes that there was no other way he could be forced to pay attention: "If I hadn't had the stroke and had to slow down, I probably would have worked myself to death." Bob is a lawyer who has been married twenty years and has two grown children. When he had his stroke, he had two small businesses in two cities and was feeling burned out. He worked hard and played hard. Relaxation was not in his vocabulary. He had had a complete medical work-up and stress test two months before the stroke and had been given a clean bill of health. There were no warning signs—no urgent messages to slow down—that is, until the stroke occurred!

In many ways, the stroke was also a blessing for Rod. Though at twenty he was younger than most of the other stroke survivors, he also may have been overcommitted to work and other pursuits. The stroke served as a wake-up call for him to reexamine his priorities. In particular, the enormous support he received from his family and friends reminded him of the importance of personal relationships. In retrospect, Rod believes he was on the edge of choosing a life that would have led him away from important life values and family-based ethics. The stroke moved him back to a life-style in which respect for other people is central and in which he could devote his life to human service.

What then is to be learned about the precursors to strokes? While many more definitive studies need to be done, our preliminary findings suggest a close connection may exist between stress and the occurrence of strokes. Further, we have found that during the period of recovery, stroke survivors must come to terms with the stressors that may have helped initiate the stroke. Survivors need to *learn* from their own past, rather than *blame* themselves for their previous mistakes (adding further to the stress). We can't change how we conducted ourselves in the past; however, like Bob, we can reinterpret the stroke as an earnest message about our priorities and responsibilities and about the level at which we conduct our daily activities. Some of us, like Bob, may need to slow down, while others, like Eldon and Jane, should recover some of the exciting and meaningful challenges that we abandoned in our effort to "slow down" or "act our age."

3

Where Am I?

I (Rod McLean) think it was fairly early in the day—whatever day it was, I didn't know. "Where am I? This isn't my bed at my house!" I looked around and saw a bunch of hospital-type things—bedtable, vinyl chair, bedcurtain, bedpan. I scanned the room. Something was not right—I was seeing everything double. I looked to my left and there was another bed. In it was a wizened-looking old man with ten to fifteen blue, red, and green plastic tubes—most of them an inch wide—all around his head, with one tube ending at an opening in the center of his throat. "Who is he?" As I glanced away, I felt disoriented and a bit apprehensive. I looked around again trying to find anything tangible to relate to, so I could figure out why I was here.

But I realized that my thinking process wasn't working the way that it usually did; the brain cells and synapses weren't poppin' as usual. Things seemed fuzzy. I very slowly calculated, "Well . . . I think this is a hospital; if it is, . . . there must be a nurse here . . . someplace? . . . I want to find out what's going on!" As I tried to roll out of the high hospital bed, my left leg kicked over the right so that both legs would be positioned to enable me to land on both feet when I bounced out of bed to retrieve a nurse. During the milliseconds involved in the "rolling-out" process, I noticed that the right leg was dragging. The leg wasn't working at all! As a matter of fact, the whole right side of my body was not moving the same way it had when I'd gotten out of bed millions of times before. And as I slid out of the bed and approached the floor, my right foot wasn't "there" when it was supposed to be. I thought

I was stepping forward toward the door, but the foot didn't take the stride and I collapsed.

As soon as I realized I was on the floor rather than about to walk through the door, I looked around from the linoleum. "I'm not supposed to be here!" Stopping for a moment to collect myself, I started noticing that I was kinda lying on my right side, flat on the floor. "Okay, I'll just prop myself with my right arm and hand. Wait a second!" I glanced at my arm, which looked strange. I knew it was mine because it was attached to my shoulder; otherwise I wouldn't have recognized it as mine. Quickly, I glanced at my right leg, too. It was in an odd position. It didn't seem to be mine either. And both limbs were flaccid, apparently without any signs of life. "What's going on here?!" I continued trying to prop my right arm up. The right arm and hand wouldn't do the task, so I even grasped the right forearm by the left hand and placed it so that I could lean on it, but it collapsed time after time. Being frightened, my brain grasped for reasons. "They must just be asleep. I must have been sleeping on them. . . ."

My fears mounted. I couldn't understand what was happening. I was racking my brains, using all my powers to reach any understanding of this new reality. There were no answers. "What's going on, Rod? Either my logic isn't working (which is very possible!), or this experience is in new territory." I just didn't seem to have any control of the right side of my body. If you could have witnessed the scenario: There I was, lying on my right side, trying to use all my strength to press up away from the cold, ammonia-scented, scrubbed floor, but to no avail. I was getting extremely frustrated; my brain was demanding that the muscles function, but nothing was reacting. "Let's stop for a minute. If those muscles don't work . . . Let's check . . . yes, the left side works! So, what the heck do I do? Let's try rolling over. Then I'll swivel and lean onto the left side."

While I was leaning and sweating I felt overwhelmed by unanswered questions. As I was realizing the depth of my dilemma, I was distracted; somebody had just walked in. "God, I hope you have some explanations and can do something about this scary situation!" My thoughts immediately reached for help from the first person I'd seen since I'd woken up: "This must have been a bad dream . . . right?" I looked up to a person wearing a white, crisp nurse's uniform. She exclaimed, "Rod, what happened? Let me help you back into your bed." I was so angry that my body just wasn't working when my brain was commanding it to do things; it wasn't cooperating. As she reached around my torso and lifted me up, I tried to assist her by pushing myself up, too. But I realized that the muscles on my right side still weren't going to allow movement. I tried to look over her left arm and shoulder at my right side so that I might see why this was happening. She swiveled me around onto the bed and pulled the cover over me, then gave me a tap on the shoulder, saying, "Glad you're awake. I'll tell the doctor and your family."

As I was attempting to concentrate and understand what she was saying, I was distracted by something very odd. Something *else* was wrong. When I looked at the nurse, I only saw half of her. "It's like I looked into her eyes, but I only saw one side. And, at the same time, I saw two images of her—one was stable, the other was just kind of floating around. As she walked out of the room, I tried looking around. I realized that I saw everything double. And when I focused on something, I only saw to my left.

So, I was going to ask her why I was there as well as many other questions. As usual, I just opened my mouth for the questions to naturally roll forth. It didn't happen! All I was able to utter was an odd-sounding jumble. "What's this?" In my head, I knew what I wanted to say, but it didn't come out right. I tried it again . . . and again . . . and again. I tried all the ideas I could think of to express my questions. Nothing worked! Am I in "Rod's twilight zone" where everything is messed up—where everything within me is distorted, crazy, disjointed, disconnected from the normal world? What made it even crazier is that everything outside and around me appeared perfectly normal, whereas everything inside me was shattered and deranged and made no sense. I didn't understand this at all. I was going to explore it all further, but I was really terrified because I didn't have control over anything.

The only thing I could really say I was certain of was that I was alive. "But wait a moment, I might be wrong!" My mind whirred in an effort to connect and correlate with anything that would make any sense at all, but nothing kicked into focus. I noticed that my thinking wasn't working the regular way. I was trying to think of something specific, but the thoughts kept eluding me. After a while, I realized that I had been fading in and out of sleep. I now realize that I had touched death and that my body's systems had experienced a major trauma. Everything had been stretched to the limit in order to keep me alive. I survived. I had been involved in a touch-and-go process, with my body trying to determine if it would live or die during that twenty-one-day coma.

So, just after I had regained consciousness, I was trying to grasp aliveness and alertness in order to survive. I was trying to use all of my capacities, even though I was running on less than half my cylinders. My consciousness was pushing all the systems' buttons, even though most of them were burned out. I faded out. I was awakened by some noises. My whole family was in front of me. I was so happy to see them. Finally! I was so glad to see someone or something that I could relate to. But as I looked at them, something odd showed on their faces. They weren't afraid or repelled; maybe it was hesitation or concern, or maybe they were not sure what to expect. It was as though I was looking through a wide-angle or even a fish-eye lens and seeing all of my family staring down at me to see if I was still me. But the experience reiterated what I'd experienced so far since I woke up—something was really off center, and I guess I was the focus of their anxiety.

When my eyes and smile showed that I was alive and conscious, my whole family burst en masse into embracing, crying, and showing love. What a feeling, knowing that my caring family was my backbone of support! In my family, everyone is so different in many ways. But when everyone was concerned with the well-being of another family member, they were there with unconditional love! Not much more can be asked. I definitely had a lump in my throat. Then I tried to express feelings and ask questions, but again the senseless "noise" came out of my mouth. I tried again, slowly reaching for the specific words that I knew were right there on the tip of my tongue. But I lost them. I was frustrated, angry, and embarrassed. I looked into their eyes for acceptance.

I laboriously formed my mouth to try speaking again, but nothing worked. Everyone either said or implied, "It's all right, Rod. Don't worry." Some of my brothers started making little jokes to lighten the mood (and to avoid their own feelings about my predicament, which is one of the ways many people deal with stressful situations).

With the ice having been broken, everyone eased into the comfort zone (me, too!). I felt secure enough to fall back to sleep. When I was first "back in the world," my main functions were sleeping, trying to eat, visiting with my many supporters, and "spacing out." My forte was sleeping. Most of the time during the next three or four days, I faded in and out of consciousness.

My family was wonderful! They either came visiting individually or together, but someone was there constantly. They were never condescending; they always led with their hearts and just accepted me. As time passed and because of their acceptance of me and my new circumstances, I could slowly begin the long, difficult process of accepting myself. My friends also saw me as "Rod," not "the new crip." All the time my family or friends were there, I tried like heck to speak (with no results). Consciously, I tried to communicate and relate to whatever was going on. Unconsciously, I tried so hard to connect with the world's reality—to try to be assured that I was still a person and to grasp for support because I was so afraid. And I wanted to use the external factors as vehicles to get out of my new, crazy world, where nothing seemed to work properly anymore. When I was awake, I constantly struggled to understand my situation. I tried to analyze, assess, and evaluate my options. Unfortunately, this was much too scary. I had to shift into my logical mind-set (which had been my strongest way of confronting problems), to test my armor, to check and see if I was still the same Rod, and to see if I was still able to use these abilities.

My thought processes were slow, mixed up, and disorganized. Demanding thoughts or ideas were "coming up on my personal computer screen," but there was a major glitch. A computer crash was about to occur. One day, I was trying to ask a friend an intricate and sophisticated question that I had been grappling with for hours. I ended up mumbling some sounds, but my friend did understand and gave a simple answer. I was surprised that I hadn't been able to figure it out and asked myself, "Is this what it's like to be mentally retarded? The brain just moves so slowly, doesn't grasp abstract concepts, and lacks the ability needed for simple understanding. Is that ever humbling! Especially when I have always relied on my intellect." This experience gave me a reference point—a taste of reality—that I didn't really want.

Since I had come out of the coma, I had just been lying in bed. Actually, I had been in that position for about a month. My mind was clear enough that I could wonder about my body's paralysis. In the past, my muscles always did what they were supposed to do: walk, run, jump, throw, catch, write, pull, push, twist—every possible motion, even down to the most minute functions, like flicking, poking, tapping—unbelievable! But if a person has never lost those functions, they just don't have a complete picture of what it's like. They can read about it or observe someone else going through it and think they know everything possible about it, but the deep core of it can only touch the soul of the individual who has actually had the intrusive experience.

After some days of just lying there being everything I could be at my basic survival level, I had collected as much data as I could. As I was reviewing the stroke's damage, I glanced at my flaccid and useless appendage, which was my seemingly dead right arm. It was strange that this arm was a part of me, for it certainly didn't seem to be. Maybe this was because there was no muscle control at all. Up until almost a month ago, everything in my being was connected and directed by my all-controlling brain. But not now! As I was staring at my useless arm, reality seeped into my consciousness: "If my mind, body, and communication systems don't function now, what's my future going to be like? It looks impossible."

At that point, I was edging down into depression. I looked back on my life: "I thought poorly about myself prior to the stroke. I was messing up in everything I touched at that time in the departments of self-image, self-development, career, the military, personal relationships, and finances." I mulled over my situation further: "If I was screwing up so much already when I was 'normal,' how could I do anything but fail now that all of my faculties aren't working? I mean, half of my body doesn't work at all, and I can't speak except for mumbling some useless sounds. My thought process is shattered and I'm scared and I have no idea what I should do. In this condition, I can't take care of myself. How can I take on so many impossible tasks? My great family will have to help me all the time . . . I can barely feed myself . . . who can help me to the bathroom? . . . family or friends will have to take me to the store or whatever . . . am I going to be bedridden forever? . . . am I going to be in a wheelchair from now on? . . . even if I get out of the house, what for? . . . my God, I won't be able to drive my car! . . . they probably won't allow me to keep my license . . . how can people listen to me when I can't talk? . . . how can they accept me? . . . after a while, I'll become nothing but a burden . . . my family and friends will quickly get bored . . . I'll lose all my friends, even the closest ones . . . oh my God!, I'll lose my fiancée, too! . . . my world will be shattered! My soul will be destroyed!"

As I was still staring at my worthless arm, my eyes filled with tears (I don't even remember how many years it had been since I had cried— macho man that I was). I was succumbing to the downside of reality, deeply depressed and swirling down the self-pity whirlpool. I was hurting. I was blaming everything on my sleeping arm and hand, when all of a sudden, my middle finger twitched! "It's alive!" With skyrocketing excitement, I quickly looked upward and in my mind said, "Thanks for this one, God!" Perfect timing. I had almost lost it. I learned that there wasn't room for self-pity. Everything in my life is up to me! And the only acceptable direction to move in was forward. That was the key. With that realization, my attitude began to change. I was gaining control of the situation. I didn't know where things were going to go, other than up. The road looked impossible, but in the back of my head, I knew everything would turn out all right.

When one confronts the reality of death, one instantly becomes humble and respectful of death as well as life. That experience leads to a soothing feeling, and it also causes a person to reprioritize the important things. My mind was suggesting that no matter what, I was still okay. Someplace in my brain was the seed of recovery; as long as I was constantly trying to get better, I would never stop and never give up.

Another realization was that life is a constant developmental process and that in actuality, the nature or severity of a person's dilemma or problem doesn't matter. What does matter is the actions one takes in response to it.

What was I going to do about my own situation? First, I set my sights on the goal and determined to go forward. I knew this was a new experience; therefore, there would be a lot of trial and error. Everything connected with the future appeared so strange and difficult. However . . . as I looked at my arm again, I asked myself, "How was I able to accomplish that twitch? Let's do it again." I constantly commanded the finger to move for maybe twenty minutes. Finally, it didn't twitch—it moved a bit to the side! "All right! Now I'm making progress!" I kept practicing for a while and became more and more excited. Ron, a close friend, walked in and saluted to get my attention, because, I guess, I was concentrating so intensely on my immediate task. As I looked at him, I beamed with excitement for accomplishing this huge (but actually minute) finger movement. I tried again and again to explain what I had done! The words just wouldn't come out. My mind was racing to find a way to explain what I had done! Again, the words wouldn't come out right. I glanced and pointed in the direction of my right hand. He was trying to figure it out, and in a moment, my formerly lifeless right finger moved again; then he understood. He shared in my excitement. What a thrill! After a while, he had to leave. But I continued to practice. "Let's try another finger . . . how about my forearm? . . . the whole arm, maybe? . . . how about the thigh or foot?" My motivation was flying! "I don't know where I'm going to end up, but this is so exciting!"

I showed the nurse what I'd accomplished, and with a smile she honestly acknowledged my first rehabilitation milestone. I guess she informed the doctor, because the next day they wheeled me down the corridor to physical therapy (at that time, I had no concept of what that might be). As we arrived, the nurse who "delivered" me loudly introduced me to the therapist. The therapist said "Hi!" in a friendly voice. She paused while she looked at the clipboard. "Rod?" I just nodded. She scanned the clipboard again, then asked a few simple questions.

I tried answering several times without success. Every time I began to reach what I wanted to say, it seemed to disappear; the more I tried, the more impossible it was to find the words. I was not only frustrated but embarrassed by exhibiting a handicap or flaw to a woman (oh, you macho man!). She acknowledged my communication dysfunction without judgment or condescension, which could have really hurt my fragile ego.

She explained that she wanted to check the status of my limbs and formulate a plan for beginning the rehabilitation process. I remember that she took my right hand and positioned it, palm up, on my right thigh. She placed a tennis ball in my palm and said, "Try to squeeze it." Her command caught me off guard. I responded by gulping and then began sweating. I quickly glanced at her and then stared at that flaccid hand. "Can I do it?" I thought up various excuses for why I couldn't but decided there was no way out. I had to do my best. I kept staring at the hand and for the longest time visualized the fingers beginning to move toward and close on that sphere, until I felt its surface. Then I felt the pressure of resistance from the seemingly cement ball. I continued staring, increasing my intensity. I started visualizing and then actually felt my muscles flex and contract. I saw the individual muscles move! The muscles of my whole body were tightening and clenching while I focused on those fingers.

After minutes had passed, I was excited to see that my middle finger and forefinger had made a minute dent in that darn tennis ball! "Whew! I guess that's how I'm gonna have to do it all the way through the process of putting myself back together." At a certain point, I felt I was at my limit and had to stop. I looked at the therapist. She acknowledged my accomplishment, saying, "That's all for right now. I'm glad to meet you, Rod." She wheeled me back to the intensive care unit; in leaving me, she gave me the tennis ball. "Don't stop," she said. "No, I won't!" I answered silently.

(Note: I won't describe all the remarkable experiences I had after my stroke in detail. By singling out a few experiences, I'm trying to show that when a person is grabbing for life and is in a survival mode, everything is overwhelmingly important. Little things loom large.)

Here are a few more pivotal experiences. During the week or so following the stroke, my family and friends came quite often. Their support was crucial. They were my lifeline when things seemed hopeless—especially when I was in a funk and couldn't muster the motivation to face all the hurdles I was facing. They gave me the boost I needed. Even though people came to visit hundreds of times, I don't remember much of what we talked about (they talked and I just tried to). But I do remember vividly that everyone who came gave me what I needed, which was just to have them there with their caring hearts.

During my two-week stay in intensive care, practically every time a nurse came to check on either me or the other patient in the room, I pleadingly asked, "What happened to me?" or "Why am I here?" In hindsight, I know that their intentions were good. However, at the time I was frustrated and angry because they would avoid eye contact with me or seemed to be preoccupied with their own thoughts to the point that they avoided confronting me. It was as if they just couldn't understand what I was trying to ask. Or, if they did understand, perhaps they would have said they were under the doctor's orders not to discuss my case with me.

I was fuming. Even then, before self-advocating was a well-known concept, I was demanding, "Look, nurse! Tell me what you know about what happened to me, so I can figure out what to do about it!" And when my doctor would come back to check on me during his rounds, he wouldn't make eye contact either. He would walk in, glance at my medical report on the clipboard and mutter to himself, put the clipboard back on the hook, and turn around and leave. Those few seconds felt like an eternity. I waited again and again for the chance to confront the doctor to find out what had happened. I often built up so much anxiety that I became even more disoriented—so much so that communication became impossible (even with myself). I felt I had the right to learn of my situation. Nowadays, this is called *self-empowerment*. Even though most likely a family member or friend did tell me the cause of my condition earlier, I don't remember being told until about two months after I was released from the hospital. I was visiting my best friend, Gary. I remember very well because when I asked him, his response was, "A stroke, of course. Hasn't anyone told you that?" At that time, I thought back and replied, "No!" No one told me or explained to me about my stroke for about a quarter of a year, and the only reason I was told was because I kept asking until someone would. The health care system does not make it easy for stroke survivors to feel empowered. You must demand or take the power for yourself! I don't mean for anyone to reject a health care professional's services or input, but the survivors should direct the plans and take part in the construction of the "new you."

I have several other strong memories of the first couple of weeks of recovery. I tried again and again to watch television, but I saw everything double. I badly wanted to watch some specific shows (subconsciously wanting to grasp another slice of "normality"). My body reacted by falling back asleep to avoid anything stressful.

An embarrassing experience occurred late one afternoon while I was still in intensive care. About five to seven friends and three or four family members were sitting or standing around my bed, talking with me or with each other. All of a sudden, I was distracted by my intestines and my anal sphincter—it was time! "Shit! (literally), what am I supposed to do? This is an emergency! Let me see . . . yes, there's no question that I have to go to the bathroom right now!"

All these people were all around me. I either had to go to the bathroom located right outside the door to the room or get the bedpan on the small table to my right. I couldn't get to the bedpan by myself; I had to ask the person closest to it to hand it to me. My voice cut through the small conversations around me. Everyone focused on me. They were surprised to hear me trying to speak and especially to hear the piercing tone of my voice: "I . . . I want . . . uh . . . uh . . . I believe . . . shit!" I was feeling under strain. I was trying to do all this stuff at the same time: not defecate in my hospital gown (which was about to occur within seconds), get the bedpan (which I really wouldn't have known how to operate), and explain to everyone that I needed the bedpan and some privacy.

All the people there recognized that I needed something; they tried to figure out my needs. They tried to read my facial language. I was grimacing, trying to control my sphincter and trying to explain the immediacy of my needs. Everyone leaned closer to understand better. "Please, help . . . shit! . . . I need bed . . . you know . . . bed, now . . . uh . . . uh . . . bed." I tried looking at the bedpan again and again. Everyone was glancing quizzically at each other, looking back at me, and guessing at what I was trying to say. It was as if we were playing charades. Look at the scenario. There I was, trying to control the uncontrollable. My eyes were turning brown. I tried to plead for the bedpan about five feet away, and my closest dozen or so friends and relatives were trying their best to help by playing charades to pull forth two of the simplest words in the English language: *bed* and *pan*!

Finally, my sphincter couldn't hold it back and I was forced to just let it rip! The stress and frenzy showing on my face were completely relieved. As a matter of fact, it wasn't as bad as I anticipated, except that I was extremely embarrassed to defecate in front of everyone. For a millisecond, everyone was huddled closely in front of me and still attempting to determine my dilemma. They couldn't understand why I suddenly wasn't concerned anymore. Immediately, they smelled the results, and everyone looked at the stainless steel bowl and said in unison, "bedpan!" They looked at each other and chuckled to break the ice. After a moment, someone went to get a nurse. And I started getting angry because I didn't like my new world. "I haven't shit in my pants since I was eighteen months old, and I hate it when I not only want to, but also *need* to talk! Damn!"

Another memory was one in which my dad came and brought a toothbrush and a razor for me. Much later, I think someone in occupational therapy suggested these activities to initiate my "self-help" tasks. Dad and the nurse helped me into the wheelchair and motored me over to the sink and the mirror. My father briefly explained that we were going to do manly things and were going to see if I could get shaved today. Then he scrubbed the lather up. Right before he was going to apply the lather, I glanced into the mirror: "Oh, my God! Who is this? Wait a minute . . . look at the eyes! Yeah, I guess it's me, but who shaved my head? And, at least as important, where'd my mustache go?" There were a couple weeks' worth of facial stubble, but no full mustache. As

I continued assessing what had happened to my face, I eventually noticed something new on the left side of my recently shaved head. While I was staring at this huge, raw, grotesque semicircular scar from the temple to behind the ear, I was wondering, "What happened to me?" And then, I gasped, "This scar is the key to what actually happened!"

I was beginning to understand the reasons why nothing on my right side was functioning properly and the reasons for my feeling crazy. This recognition allowed me to begin accepting myself as not being the cause of the problem; the mirror had provided a link with the "real" world. Then I looked at Dad. He acknowledged that I was ready to at least attempt shaving—but not the mustache, a part of my old identity that was gone! It was the first time I had shaved left handed. It all seemed so difficult, just as if I were attempting this task for the first time. I guess I didn't do too terribly; I only ended up with five bloody nicks. My family saw me gazing into the mirror, totally mesmerized by the scar and the shaved head. Then someone (a family member or nurse) came up with the brilliant idea of applying a puke-green hospital cap to my head; it had little ties that secured the bonnet under the chin. "Cute, huh? Now I can tell that I'm a real patient." It was interesting that I was allowed to continue wearing the cap, maybe because it was "doctor's orders."

Another discovery reflected in the mirror was that I seemed thinner than before. At some point during my mother's many visits, she mentioned that I'd lost thirty-five pounds while comatose; at that time, I was fed intravenously. When I began to recover, I was constantly hungry. Every mealtime, no matter what was presented to me, I would gobble up every bit of the repast (even the vegetables I had never liked before). I mean, I was so hungry that I even thought that the notorious cafeteria-style hospital food was "Top of the Mark" (my compliments to the chef!). To me, being able to eat and feed myself were pivotal accomplishments: by again doing basic things like that, I was regaining some control over my life. During the task of relearning how to feed myself like a toddler, I fumbled with the fork, trying to scoop or stab at the gourmet vittles and raise them to my mouth. I even tried to recreate the chewing process. I felt so inadequate. It was a humbling experience—a shot of reality.

I remember that when I awoke from the coma and started realizing that something major had happened to me, the first question that came to mind was, "Can I still have sex?" I was fairly sexually active and my sexual identity was extremely important to me. Since I came out of the coma, Linda, my fiancée, had offered her support by visiting me at the hospital many times. She acted just the way she should within the context of our relationship. There were flowers, visits, sweet talk, hand-holding. Many people had come visiting the third postcoma evening for a great old time. After everyone except Linda left, I was feeling so happy having such great parents, siblings, and friends. After a few moments, she toned down the lights, and her soft kisses changed the mood. She slid onto the tall hospital bed, hugged me, and snuggled into her regular position in our "old" embrace.

It was terrific! I started to feel as though I was in a groove; I was exhilarated. I felt my "powers" coming back! I started feeling normal. "But wait! I don't know . . . I'm all messed up now. I can't talk, my brain and the right side of my body don't work . . . I wonder? . . . does my sexual plumbing still work?" Instantly, I experienced a feeling of shock and of being frozen by the possibility of the unknown. I was totally afraid that my tools didn't function . . . "Oh, Linda, I'm not sure if . . ." Twangg! " . . . Whew! Something down there's rustling." I felt better but still scared. "There are so many things to be found out."

About a week after I awoke from the coma, my whole family came not only to visit, but also to take me to a different hospital in Puyallup, Washington. They told me that I'd improved enough to go to a rehabilitation hospital. I really wasn't sure what that might be. When the family arrived, though, they were really upbeat, and so their feelings gave me a good charge of hope for the future. I was making tangible progress. After everyone joked around for a couple of minutes, the nurse came in and rolled the wheelchair to the side of my bed. The family kind of just fell into motion preparing to leave, and said, "Well, let's go!" I beamed with excitement. I didn't really know where I was going, but my attitude and psyche were set in the direction of getting out of there. I wanted to go anywhere to get away from this insane dilemma! And if my family was happy and looking forward to the change, it must be good.

The nurse approached to help me into the wheelchair. I looked at her, resisted, and tried to verbalize that I was going to do it by myself. I concentrated in an effort to use all my muscles to transfer from the bed to the wheelchair. It looked so precarious. I thought squeezing that tennis ball was so difficult because I had to use five or ten muscles, whereas right then, I had to try to coordinate all my muscles—even the ones that worked. Not only that, but I had to balance my asymmetrical body as I descended into the wheeled contraption that I was seeing two of due to my double vision. "Whew! I made it! Now I had to rearrange my gown. But wait a second! If I was supposed to go someplace, shouldn't I have gotten dressed? Where were my clothes? And was I going to have to dress myself?"

My father stepped forward with a shopping bag full of clothes. He glanced at the nurse, questioning whether to help me, and if so, how? I think my face showed that I was stuck. "What do I do now?" Instantly, I felt shocked and angered that I was without options and that I had to rely on others. "Okay, I'll succumb. What do I have to do? Show me and let's do it." The nurse told me how to get back on the bed, gave me the clothes, and explained how to start dressing with the pants, shirt, and so on. She let me try my new tasks, helping me when necessary. "I feel so dumb and handicapped! This is all baby stuff! I guess I really am messed up."

4

Confronting
Reality

Sheila's initial experience after having regained consciousness following her stroke closely resembles that of Rod McLean—and many other stroke survivors we interviewed. She first realized that something was different about her body when she tried to get out of her hospital bed to use the restroom. She fell twice and stayed on the floor, realizing her body would not cooperate with her thoughts. Sheila then made an attempt to ask a nurse questions and was shocked to hear her jumbled words. Lying on the floor and urinating on herself, Sheila vividly recalls feeling profoundly humiliated.

This is a critical phase—the first phase—in the process of recovering from a stroke. For Sheila, Rod, and other stroke survivors, it is a time filled with fear, pain, and attempts to come to grips with reality. What has happened to me and what will become of me? These are the two critical questions survivors initially confront. In this chapter, we begin by exploring the first question and address the issue of being informed about having had a stroke. We then turn to the second question and consider the immediate physical implications of the stroke—as reflected in the physical therapy survivors must undergo—and then the longer-term implications regarding changes in self-image, relationships, and life-style.

What Has Happened to Me?

One of the most shocking findings of our study was the failure of health care professionals to make information available to stroke survivors immediately after their stroke. As Rod noted in his account, doctors and nurses often do not bother to inform the survivors of what occurred, or if they do inform them, it is done in a manner or at a time when they cannot comprehend or remember the information. When John awoke in the hospital, he suspected that he had had either a heart attack or a stroke. It was several hours before he saw the doctor, and when he finally did, John recalled that the doctor was rushed and generally unpleasant. For several days, John was not told what had happened to him, nor did he receive any information regarding his current health. Finally, the doctor came into John's room and said that he believed that John was malingering and asked if he was receiving any sort of psychological counseling. John was astounded that the doctor had even suggested this, given that he continued to have difficulties speaking, moving his left side, and remembering names of friends. Other doctors later confirmed that John had in fact had a stroke.

While doctors in contemporary hospitals are under considerable stress and it is understandable that they have little time to spend with each patient, it is also critical to note that those initial contacts between the stroke survivor and physician often have a dramatic and lasting impact on the survivor's perceptions of his or her prospects for recovery. Even more basically, these initial contacts between doctor and patient help to define the survivor's sense of self-confidence and self-esteem. At this early, critical phase, the survivor has just begun the long process of reconstructing the psychological as well as physical well-being that was abruptly taken away at the moment the stroke took place. Health care professionals must assist or at least not retard this process.

At least one professional in the hospital should be responsible for providing stroke survivors with information about what happened to them. When a rehabilitation counselor or social worker meets with stroke survivors and their families, they should give them a substantial amount of educational material, yet must also help them make sense of this material, so that they are not overwhelmed. The American Heart Association has put together a packet of information on resource material for stroke survivors, a booklet on aphasia (impairment of the ability to use or understand speech), a booklet on how left- and right-side brain damage affects behavior, and a booklet on the risk factors and warnings signs of stroke. These highly readable documents are obtainable from the American Heart Association and should be available at any hospital or rehabilitation center that serves stroke survivors. Stroke survivors and caregivers should also typically be given a nutritional guide and information on a low-fat/low-cholesterol diet to encourage prevention of future strokes and to give these people something tangible they can do in response to the difficult situation they face.

We also suggest that stroke survivors and caregivers be given a videotape titled *The Brain at Risk,* which is out of print but available at hospitals and rehabilitation centers. This video explains three types of strokes: thrombotic, embolic, and hemorrhagic—and is a wonderful tool to help families and survivors identify the warning signs of these afflictions and the risk factors associated with them. The tape also identifies ways stroke survivors can change their behavior to avoid future strokes. Most families check this video out of hospitals over a weekend. They are encouraged to watch the videotape together, so that they can discuss the implications of the information it presents for each family member.

Unfortunately, not all health care professionals seem to be concerned about getting information to stroke survivors and their families—even the basic information that they have had a stroke. In counseling sessions, we are confronted time and time again with the recurring story of survivors not being given this information or other, more specific information, such as on what type of stroke has occurred. We are repeatedly amazed not only at this uncaring behavior on the part of professionals, but also at their failure to encourage survivors to progress and heal. Because of the pervasiveness of these incidents, it is essential that professional caregivers have physicians (neurologists in particular) present an in-service training program on strokes for members of stroke support groups. Professional caregivers should also provide members of these groups with up-to-date information on new techniques in preventing or diagnosing strokes.

Grace was one of the unfortunate stroke survivors who was told virtually nothing about her stroke, either immediately after she woke up or at a later time. Like Rod, she was perplexed by the absence of information when she regained consciousness. She was finally told about having a stroke, but only hours after arriving at the hospital. "This was weird, you know," observes Grace. "I would like to have known right away. The sooner you do something about something, the better off you are." She went on to concede that the physicians and nurses "know more than I do" about what they ought to be doing. Nevertheless, she thought that it was "strange not to know what was wrong with me. No one wanted to tell you. I had no idea. All I knew was that all I wanted to do was sleep." She also noted—as did most of the people we interviewed—that no one at the hospital worked with her specifically with regard to the psychological implications of the stroke. Rather, they spoke about her in her presence as if she weren't there and didn't need information about what had occurred in her life.

Even when the physicians and nurses told relatives of the stroke survivors about the stroke and its implications, this information was often not conveyed to the survivors themselves. Alice remembers nothing from before, during, or after the stroke. She was told she was in the hospital immediately after having her stroke but can remember nothing. She described the experience as one of waking up from a bad dream. She was in the hospital for about a week and did not know why she was there or why she was taken away from her home. Alice indicated that she "started having weird thoughts . . . you know . . . like why did they put me here." She heard her husband talk about the stroke but still did not know what it was or what the symptoms were.

To provide a balanced picture, we should note that some stroke survivors received wonderful treatment from their physicians. Margaret spoke of receiving a substantial amount of immediate and continuing support from her large family, physician, and other caregivers. Her physician immediately saw her after her fall, told her that she probably had a stroke, and ordered extensive testing. Twelve family members came to the hospital that morning and got a full report on her condition from the doctor. He gave her and her family a clear, specific, and lengthy report on the tests when the results were available—though she couldn't remember the details at the time she was interviewed.

Like Margaret, Georgia had a very positive experience: "It took me a while after the shock [of having a stroke] to understand what had happened to me. The doctors explained to me what happened and my daughters also did." She noted that

> the doctors were very kind and sympathetic with me and my family. They explained to me and my family what to expect as far as progress with my health [was concerned]. They told me what kinds of changes to expect in the coming year. They taught me about nutrition. I used to be a red meat eater but since my stroke I don't eat meat at all. I have turned into a vegetarian. I was told to continue speech therapy. I was in the hospital for two and one-half months. Six months after my stroke, I was speaking again. The doctors told me I was progressing really well.

Margaret and Georgia were fortunate to receive the careful attention they did from their physicians. Both of these women (and their relatives) were provided with accurate and useful information about the stroke. Georgia's physician, furthermore, spoke with her about the changes she could anticipate in her life during the coming year, without making her feel that these changes were inevitable or permanent. Her doctor also offered her specific suggestions concerning ways to avoid future strokes and ways to recover lost functions. These four areas of assistance seem to be critical to successful recovery from strokes: (1) valid and useful information about the stroke itself, (2) valid and useful—though nonbinding—information about conditions that might be realistically expected during the year(s) immediately following the stroke, (3) valid and useful information about ways to avoid strokes in the future, and (4) valid and useful information about resources that can be relied on in recovering from strokes.

This information must be provided not only to stroke survivors but also to relatives and caregivers. It must often be delivered repeatedly in a clear and simple manner that takes into account the survivor's possibly disrupted memory and related cognitive functions, and that takes into account the anxiety, confusion, and anger experienced by the survivor and relatives immediately following the stroke. Margaret received a full report, yet, as we noted, very little of this report registered with her in the early stages of the recovery process. Beth remembered that her doctor came into her room when she awoke after her stroke and told her that she was "fortunate" she'd had a minor stroke rather than a heart attack. With a tone of confusion in her voice, Beth indicated that she still doesn't understand what the doctor meant when he told her she was lucky. Beth expressed much sadness about the permanency of the effects of her stroke and finds it difficult to identify herself as "lucky."

Susan woke up after three weeks in a coma. She said that "with God's grace, I was spared awareness of the actual event. I remember standing up and everything went black." She woke up in the hospital three weeks later, her husband, children, mother, and physician being in attendance. Her doctor attempted to explain her condition, but she couldn't relate to it at all. Compounding this problem is the frequent inability of stroke survivors to communicate their frustration about not being told or not being able to understand what is being said. Many survivors share with Rod the exasperating experience of trying to let their doctor, nurse, or relative know that they want to be informed or missed what was just said. However, they must lie there passively and mute, having lost their capacity to speak. Margaret vividly recalled just such an experience: "[When I woke up in the hospital] I wanted to know where I was and no one understood me . . . I don't think I really knew what happened to me until later. I mean about being paralyzed . . . I think it was a nurse who told me that I had a stroke . . . she told me I was having a hard time making myself understood." One wonders if Margaret really had to be told that other people didn't understand her! Like others we interviewed, Margaret often received information that was absolutely useless to her. No one seems to have taken the time to put themselves in her shoes in order to determine what kind of information she might want and how best to convey this information to her. Given her inability to speak, those closest to her could no longer rely on her feedback. They needed to anticipate her needs and find ways to be particularly sensitive to any verbal or nonverbal feedback she was able to give regarding the adequacy of what she was told by the physician, nurses, or relatives.

Even when the stroke survivor and caregivers are informed about the stroke, they are often confronted briefly and ineffectively with a pessimistic prognosis that tends to leave them with a sense that they will have little to say about their recovery. Sheila said that the one thing still bothering her about the initial stroke experience is the way her doctor described her condition. Apparently, he told her that her present condition would not change. She would continue to be paralyzed on the right side and would not regain the ability to speak. "It seemed," said Sheila with considerable indignation, "that he was telling me that I didn't have anything to look forward to!" Greta similarly reported that her first experiences with her doctors, nurses, and physical therapists were upsetting because she found them to be negative about her prospects for recovery. She stated that every professional she dealt with wanted her to "accept my disability." She was told she must "live with it" and became angry and frustrated with the medical profession regarding their pervasive negativism.

Roberta received a similar dose of pessimism from the medical staff at the hospital where she was treated following her stroke. She was unaware of what had happened to her when she awoke in the hospital but was soon told that she had a stroke and was in a coma for forty-eight hours. Furthermore, she was told that she was paralyzed on the right side of her body. To combat this paralysis, she began an extensive rehabilitation program during the following seven weeks at the hospital. Roberta engaged in physical therapy, some of which consisted of physical training in a swimming pool three times per week. She learned to use a wheelchair in three weeks. She then learned how to walk with a cane.

Throughout this successful rehabilitation, Roberta was advised by the hospital staff that she would never fully recover from her stroke. However, she refused to accept this prediction—until she was fitted for a brace. It was only after she left the hospital that she began to confront the fact of an altered life-style. Apparently, during her stay at the hospital, she was constantly fighting the pronouncements made by the staff concerning her limitations. Her rapid rehabilitation may, in fact, have been motivated in part by her strong wish to prove the hospital staff wrong. Only after discharge from the hospital was she able to set aside her resistance and denial to confront the reality of her new, lifelong physical limitations.

Similarly, Greta resented the pessimism expressed by many staff members at the hospital. She suggested that stroke survivors need to feel hope, not discouragement. As perhaps in the case of Roberta, the anger that Greta felt regarding the staff's negativism eventually served as a motivator for her. She refused to give up, for this would have confirmed the staff members' pessimistic predictions. Initially, however, when she first faced the staff's negativism, she became depressed and felt profound hopelessness. In these early stages, she cried a great deal and was only able to overcome her depression through grief work done with a psychologist. While for Roberta, the negativism of the hospital staff may have actually been a positive motivator, one must wonder to what extent this is always the case. How many stroke survivors—like Greta—give up trying to fully recover because their doctors, nurses, and therapists offer accurate but insensitively timed statements regarding their probable future restrictions? Greta was able to convert her anger to hard rehabilitative work, but what about those stroke survivors who are unable to overcome their depression or convert their anger to commitment?

Is it really appropriate to set limits so soon in the treatment process? Isn't hope (even if somewhat unrealistic) essential to the early mobilization of physical resources for healing and overcoming at least some of the limits imposed by the stroke? As Carla mentioned, "I'm glad that at the time I didn't know that a year later I would still not be walking." A little denial and wishful thinking may be appropriate at this early stage.

We should, once again, offer a balanced perspective by describing several of those instances when health care professionals were supportive and encouraging. Tom indicated that he "had a good doctor and

I knew I was going to get well." Tom laughed at this point and exclaimed, "I guess it's a good thing I didn't know what was ahead for me." Tom said he learned nothing about his condition from his doctor—who had been a long-time family friend. He added, however, that his physician may have talked with his wife about his stroke, but he can't remember if this occurred. Tom noted that "I figured they'd tell me if I needed to know." He feels that his hospital care was good and that everyone did everything they could to help him. He was in the hospital for about three weeks and received minimal therapy. They wanted to keep him longer at the hospital, but he just wanted to get home to his garden. While Tom's physician might have kept him better informed about his physical condition and might have helped him be more realistic about the recovery process, would this really have been helpful? Wasn't it more important that Tom's physician was encouraging and left him with the sense that he was "going to get well"?

The so-called "defensive" processes of denial and unrealistic optimism are not necessarily detrimental—particularly at early stages in the recovery from a stroke. Given the frightening, all-encompassing impact of the stroke on most survivors, it is not surprising that the first thing they need is reassurance and support from someone knowledgeable and in charge: the physician. To the extent that this reassurance and support is not available, doctors are doing an inadequate job of treating the stroke survivors and of maximizing their chances for recovery.

While the stroke survivors often complained about the lack of adequate information and often-indifferent treatment from the physicians when first coming to the hospital, virtually all our informants spoke positively about the medical and physical treatment they received during their hospital stay. They talked about the competence of the nursing and physical therapy staffs and usually believed that the treatment for their physical ills was adequate. Carla expressed her appreciation for the work of one nurse who was patient and understanding when she lost control of her bowels. She had heard another nurse scold a patient in a similar situation. Others spoke similarly of patient and supportive nurses and of physical therapists who encouraged them to keep trying during their long rehabilitation efforts.

In several cases, the physical treatment program was clearly difficult for the survivors. Margaret—who had received wonderful treatment when first entering the hospital—said her speech therapist made her particularly angry when they first worked together. Over time, however, they became close; now, "she is like a daughter to me." At first, everything became "one great big pain" for Margaret, and in her disoriented mental state, she almost became unable to distinguish friend from foe: "Every time I would close my eyes someone would be there jabbing at me, encouraging me to do something . . . I just wanted to be left alone . . . I was so tired and they kept bothering me . . . everything hurt so bad and no one could understand me . . . everyone kept telling me not to be afraid . . . I wasn't afraid; I was furious . . . my head hurt so bad I thought it was splitting in two and I couldn't get anyone to understand."

While the poking and goading may have been critical to Margaret's rehabilitation, the continuing lack of information reported by some stroke survivors can never be justified, nor can the seeming indifference of some hospital staff to the difficult transition of stroke survivors back to the "real world" when they leave the hospital. Carla reported both of these failures. No one sat down to discuss the stroke with her during her two and a half months in the hospital. She indicates that she would have liked to talk to someone—"having no one to discuss it with me was the worst part." In time, she did begin to feel close to some of the staff members; however, none of them came to say good-bye when she left. When she returned to her room to say good-bye to her roommate, there was already someone in "her" bed. Carla spoke of having "a funny feeling" about this immediate replacement of herself with another person.

What Will Become of Me?

While denial and hopeful thinking may be wonderful antidotes early in the recovery process, there is a point when stroke survivors (and their caregivers) must confront at least some of the implications of the stroke for their immediate and future lives. What is the nature of this confrontation and how much assistance do stroke survivors receive when they are forced to consider often-painful implications?

Jane's stroke came as a complete surprise. She woke up in the morning at the hospital with her right side paralyzed and numb. During the subsequent three days, she experienced constant spasms that were so severe that she was unable to get any sleep. She said the spasms prevented her from confronting all the realities of having a stroke. The spasms demanded all of her attention. She was unable to think of anything else and was incapable at the time of drawing on her past life experiences to consider the severity of her situation or prospects for her future. Thus, even though other members of her family had previously had strokes, Jane was completely overwhelmed and frightened by her personal encounter with the disability and pain associated with her own stroke experience. Once the spasms subsided, however, she began to experience strong feelings: anxiety, depression, and frustration.

Though Georgia had been given ample information about her stroke and its implications, the recognition was still painful: "The first thing I thought was, I don't want to be a burden to my children. I was so depressed and upset that this happened. I didn't know what to do." Susan, by contrast, was able to make use of earlier experiences in her life in confronting the implications of her stroke. The sources of reassurance for her, however, were not necessarily reliable: "If I really had a stroke, everything will be fine because that is the way it happens in movies. The stroke victim always recovers from the event."

Clearly, considering the implications of the event is psychologically stressful. Yet if little or no time is set aside for this reflection and if psychological support is unavailable, the outcomes can be even more disturbing. John spent only a short time in the hospital after his stroke and did little reflecting on how his stroke might change his life. He gave minimal attention to ways he needed to change his relationships with others and ways he would now need support from them. He was sent home and received no professional aftercare for nearly a year. Without giving it much thought, he began to rely heavily on friends to bring him his meals and care for him. He was somewhat mobile in that with a walker, and considerable effort, he was able to take himself to the restroom. However, in many other ways he was growing increasingly dependent on other people—which he hated.

John was depressed and angry immediately following his stroke. He was hostile toward his doctor, feeling that this man lacked sensitivity and was not trustworthy. John also felt hopeless and lost any desire to care for himself. He began considering placing himself in a skilled nursing facility but dreaded the thought of this, because he knew it would mean the end of his independence. Those people who he considered his friends began coming around less frequently and—according to John—began treating him as a nuisance. Thus, at the time of the interview, John was taking a second look at the nursing home and found the prospect of receiving professional care to be logical. Perhaps some form of psychotherapy would be appropriate, given the magnitude and complexity of John's feelings regarding his stroke.

Consistently, throughout the interviews, stroke survivors indicated that not only did they not receive any psychological treatment after their stroke, but they also were rarely even told about the availability of such services. No one recommended psychological assistance to either Sheila or her family. She regrets that she and her family received no assistance. Jim also recalled no offer of psychological support, while Margaret indicated that she didn't see any need for therapy because she wasn't "crazy." However, later, when she reflected on her need for someone to talk with during this difficult period, Margaret said she wished she had gotten some of this support. She became visibly disturbed when recounting that she had received no information about the "real" nature of psychological counseling and therapy for people who aren't "crazy" but are under considerable stress.

Thelma stayed at a local hospital for a total of twelve days. She received no psychological services. No one asked her about her feelings. She told no one about her thoughts of suicide, which were quite strong. Once a day she went for occupational therapy. She reported that the therapists helped her learn how to prepare meals with one hand, but she did not feel that she received adequate help or encouragement in overcoming her paralysis—nor did anyone ask her about her feelings after such a profound experience as having a stroke and waking up paralyzed.

Thelma feels that her treatment suffered because of this total lack of responsiveness to her emotional needs. She is convinced that no one comprehended what she was going through and that most people seemed to be uncomfortable when talking with her about her stroke experience. According to Thelma, the medical staff weren't any better at handling her condition in this respect than was her husband. She suggested that the most effective treatment might have been to introduce her to other stroke survivors early in her recovery. Thelma believes that they have a "natural understanding" and a wealth of practical advice that would have made her recovery from depression much easier.

Georgia did speak with a psychologist one time because of her recurring depression. However, mostly she "prayed a lot to God." Furthermore, the priest from her church came by and talked with her, offering psychological support and counsel. Susan noted that while her doctor explained the physical ramifications of her stroke in great detail, he provided no insights concerning the psychological ramifications, nor did he recommend any counseling or psychotherapy. Susan emphasized that such treatment would have been helpful to her during the early stages of her adjustment to the stroke and said she frequently encourages other stroke survivors to receive psychological assistance.

Bob similarly reported that he received no assistance immediately following his stroke, nor during the long recuperative and rebuilding period. He now sees that he was very depressed following his stroke and that this depression lasted at least two years. According to Bob, his medical needs were attended to, but no one helped him confront his emotional needs. He is angry that not one of the medical personnel he saw ever mentioned that he might have psychological needs in dealing with his stroke. He said that "it should be part of the package, just like physical therapy."

It is clear from the interviews we reviewed that the first poststroke experiences are inevitably confusing and frightening to the survivors. Bewilderment and fear are present, even if the survivors are knowledgeable about strokes because of having previously had a stroke or because of having treated others with strokes. While these strong feelings will not go away in most cases for several weeks, the poststroke experience can become less stressful if the survivors are given information about their stroke in a clear and timely manner soon after they have regained consciousness and are no longer in great physical pain. This information should be provided to both the survivors and their caregivers. One should not assume that the job is done simply by handing it to caregivers. Stroke survivors want to hear the important details directly from someone they respect (and hopefully trust) who is a medical authority. In most cases, this person should be the physician.

Our findings also suggest that survivors need substantial reassurance, not just from their relatives and friends but also from medical professionals. This reassurance is particularly important at the point when survivors first confront the prospect of substantial changes in their lives. Medical professionals should not assume that these concerns do not emerge until the survivors are ready to leave the hospital. Most of the people we interviewed indicated that they became concerned about their future (and the future of others in their lives) immediately after they realized that they were going to survive the stroke.

The nature of the reassurance is particularly important. Health care professionals should not lie to a stroke survivor. Those we interviewed seemed to be keenly aware of it when they were not getting the truth. On the other hand, stroke survivors should be given information about their stroke in a manner that allows them the opportunity to hope. Statements delivered by health care professionals that are interpreted as pessimistic and that dismiss the survivors' ability to overcome major obstacles tend to evoke enormous hostility. This hostility does motivate some survivors to try harder. More often, however, the hostility is directed inward and leads to depression. The pessimism frequently becomes self-fulfilling. If stroke survivors are told that they have little chance to fully recover, they are likely to give up trying, thereby confirming the prediction. Health care professionals must be particularly sensitive to self-fulfilling prophecies, for we found ample evidence that this was occurring among the stroke survivors we interviewed.

What form, then, should the reassurance take? In essence, information should always be interlaced with encouragement. Stroke survivors should feel that they know what has happened to them and what possible developments might occur in the future. They want this dose of reality. In addition, however, they would like the health care authorities to mention that people do recover from strokes—even from severe strokes. Furthermore, survivors should be told that tangible evidence suggests that a positive attitude helps the healing process: in trying harder, one is actually helping to heal oneself! This message of hope tempered with realism is essential, and it must come from someone in authority, while being reinforced by friends and relatives. It is at this point that recovery begins.

PART TWO

Adapting to the Stroke

5

What's Going to Happen to Me?

We pulled up to the grounds of the rehabilitation center and were received by a candy striper with a wheelchair. She wheeled me (Rod McLean) around the corridor and up the elevator to the fourth floor. She steered the chair around and past some physical therapy and occupational therapy equipment and some other people in wheelchairs. As I was passing some of the individuals, we made eye contact and they seemed to ask, "Who is this new guy with a seven-person entourage following him toward the registration desk?"

From the moment I was wheeled out of the elevator toward the desk, I felt a whole realm of different emotions: excitement, apprehension, depression with regard to my detachment from the outside world, and anticipation that I would soon get it all back together. From the eye contact made, I immediately felt like an outsider watching these weird "cripples," but as I wheeled past them, I was frozen by the realization that I was one of them! Still, as I look back on my entire three-week stint at this rehab center, I can see that a part of me observed the whole scene from afar and remained detached from others at the center, even though I knew why I was there and did my best to accomplish my own and the center's goals. It's as if I were a fly on the wall, just watching it all.

A nurse introduced herself to me as she wheeled me to one of the bedrooms. She described the facility, its services and philosophy: "We see this as a dorm . . . we're anticipating another man to be your roommate within a week or so. You know that people come from many other states. You are lucky that your family lives so close." I nodded and smiled as I looked behind me at my family. The nurse chitchatted as she opened the bedcurtain, pointed to the bathroom, lights, and button board. She explained about the center's various departments and where they were located. These included the social area, physical therapy, occupational therapy, the counseling room, and the multiactivity room. She puttered around and stopped to look at me and said, "Rod, I'm really glad you're here and I hope things go well." And, poof, she disappeared! Not really, but it seemed so because all of a sudden and just for a moment there was silence. I think my family was stunned for a moment, too. But they soon left.

I chose the bed closest to the window and bathroom. Within a few minutes, a different nurse peeked into my "dorm" room and informed me that dinner would be served in the multiactivity room at five. "I guess I'm supposed to wheel myself to get there." As I was thinking during the process of getting ready, I glanced to the right and noticed that my hand was just dangling outside the wheelchair arm. I remembered to place my (temporarily) useless hand on my lap while I was wheeling. "Okay, I've got that, but what do I do next?" Before, I had noticed that the nurses had secured the wheelchair by locking the brakes, so I had to release them. "That's done. I guess I just wheel out of here now. Here we go . . . let's get around the foot of the bed before I attempt to exit through the door. Whoops! I thought the doorway was wide enough. Well, I guess it is, but I didn't see the doorjamb on the right side. How do I go backward? Figure it out, Rod! Hallelujah, I'm now in the hallway!"

I looked and saw two guys rolling down the hall where the light was. I thought, "I bet that's where I should be going for dinner, but I have to figure out how to get this chair from here to there." I wheeled for a while, but during every other attempt at propelling it, the right side of the wheelchair crashed against the right side of the wall! You see, I could only use my left arm to thrust this vicious projectile, so it just wouldn't stay on course. I had noticed before that there were eight-inch-wide metal strips running parallel to the floor from one end of the hall to the other; these strips were all at wheelchair height. While

I was desperately trying to move around in that uncontrollable machine and smashing into the wall, it sure seemed that the metal strips had a strong magnetism that attracted the very-metal wheelchair!

After I crashed enough times to stop and try to analyze it, I realized that most likely it wasn't really magnetic, even though it seemed so. Maybe it was because I was only able to move one wheel at a time. "Rod, why was that so hard to figure out? It's so frustrating when you know that your brain ought to be running on all cylinders! Well, I've got one hand to use but not the other. How else can I help this vehicle move, or at least find something to help me navigate a straighter course? . . . (pause) . . . (pause) . . . come on, Rod! . . . Let's use the other workable limb—my left foot! Yeah, I can try to shuffle and steer. It's taking so long and using so much energy. Let's go eat!"

It did take a while, but as I approached the dining room, I became frightened of arriving and entering the room. When I entered I would be "knighted" as one of "those" people. I was definitely feeling resistant to becoming "one of them." I thought to myself, "I completely hate this crazy world, and I don't accept the 'new' Rod. I will only accept finding the road back to where I was before I blew a gasket! Well, okay, I'm hungry. I'll try it out!" Gulp! As I entered the room, there were some glances (as well as eye contact), smiles, and acknowledgments. As one of the nurses began talking to me, I felt, "Well, these guys are just people." I let go of my shock.

The nurse introduced herself and wheeled me while suggesting that I sit at one of the four-, eight-, or ten-foot circular tables. I made a quick assessment: all men, all ages, all very different, and all used some type of contraption, the likes of which I had never seen and was unable to figure out. The nurse who escorted me to the dinner table asked me if she could assist me. I mumbled that it would be fine if she did. I expected that she would position my meal so that I could eat with my left hand or that she would serve me. Instead, she sat to my right, grasped my right hand, and slid my useless fingers into an odd-looking leather-and-metal brace to which she attached a spoon and caringly said, "Let's try some soup. It's pretty good." I looked at this thing around my hand and felt like shaking it away as if it were a scorpion or something equally grotesque.

I looked at her and tried to speak, but nothing made any sense. She looked into my eyes and said, "It's all right," and confirmed the statement with her strong eyes. I trustingly tried to ask how to use the apparatus. "Try to remember how you used to feed yourself," she said. "Try to do it again. Concentrate on using all those muscles. Squeeze your fingers as tightly as you can around that tape-wrapped spoon stem, lift up, extend forward, drop it into the bowl; lift and contract the muscles to transport the precious cargo over the (precariously positioned) bowl and help it travel to the reaching mouth." But I thought, "How do I actually do all this?"

I looked at her again, then looked at my hand and its "helper." I proceeded to concentrate as hard as I could on performing the task. I felt some energy and was aware of perspiration on my brow. The arm-hand-fingers system was trembling but nothing was really moving the way it was supposed to. "Okay, I'm really gonna focus . . . " The hand and spoon started moving! "Great! That little spoon weighs a ton—so much that I can barely lift it!" I continued glaring at it. I was surprised at how strenuous it was to initiate hoisting the spoon and, at the same time, I was so exhilarated that the dormant muscles had begun to flex! I took another deep breath and tried to move the spoon closer to the steaming bowl and then to my salivating mouth. The hand paused and shook a bit and the spoon splashed into the soup!

I stopped the concentration and repositioned the spoon with my left hand. Refocusing was needed. I then felt my shoulder rise, with my torso leaning forward. My fingers felt as if they were pinching through the apparatus to the slender metal piece that gave me access to my life-saving food. My attention was focused completely on my hand. I glanced at the tip of the spoon as it approached the lip of the bowl while I lifted it just a smidgen and dropped it into the soup (whew!). I took a quick breath, then regained the mind-set needed to once again clasp the spoon through the apparatus. But before I started lifting the spoonful of soup, I thought, "How in the devil am I going to do this? I can barely lift the spoon, but now I not only have to lift the weight, I also have to do it gently, smoothly, and with strength. Right now I have to do something that I haven't done since before the stroke a month ago, and now I know I can do it! Let's go for it!"

The gross muscles were trying to do their best to perform fine motor tasks. It was awkward and a bit jerky. Also, it was difficult to coordinate all those muscles, perform tasks requiring eye-hand coordination, and think at the same time; it was just too much for me to do. I couldn't remember it all and balance everything each individual second. The spoon had lifted about three inches above the soup, and I was pulling it toward me. The soup and spoon began quivering again, and I felt my biceps twitch and my fingers reacting. Then the spoon lost its balance and the soup splashed on the table. I looked at the nurse. She nodded and reached toward my arm to set it up again. Immediately, I responded, "I'll do it!"

I glared at my hand that had screwed up. Then I totally focused; I saw nothing but my hand, the spoon, and the soup. I visualized how it all was going to work together to get that damn soup into my mouth! I mentally went through the sequences to the point of the crash. Concentrating even more, I squeaked right past the previous problem. As my hand and gear approached the destination, I felt the muscles tightening up. They were stretching to their limits. My mouth lunged and snapped forward and clamped onto the spoon as I swallowed some of the soup and the rest dribbled down my chin. "Hooray! I was really worried. I didn't think I was capable of doing that at all. I'll have to show this to the family."

After my excitement subdued, I thought, "Do I have to do this much for each sip for the rest of my life?" Getting a glimpse of what I might have to go through really scared me! "If this minuscule task is so difficult, how about the literally millions of other things I have to do! Rod . . . hey, Rod . . . remember when you first became depressed and all of a sudden that middle finger twitched, and you absolutely put your blinders on and said you'd never give up? Don't forget that!"

When I finished the soup, I was proud to have completed the task. Not long ago I could barely hold that tennis ball in my hand; shortly before that, I had the experience with the twitching finger. It's getting better. The nurse put her hand on my shoulder and looked into my eyes, warmly conveying her approval. I responded with my crooked smile. Then, as she cleaned my messy eating place, I looked around the room and noticed all the other guys. Some were not aided by devices, but others were eating with different types of "helpers" or were being fed.

There's something for me to learn from this situation. I'm not sure what it means right now, but I'll shelve it until it makes sense." I also noticed that during and especially after finishing, a lot of conversations started all over the room—one on one, in small clusters, and everyone all together at a couple of tables. I was so startled because the first thing I saw was all these wheelchairs and gurneys and all sorts of unbelievable machines with strange gadgets. But when the talking started, I observed that there were smiles and jokes being cracked. "These 'crips' are just people. They are just *normal*! I'll be damned!"

All of a sudden, I wanted to see if I was a "cool crip." Someone at my table told a pretty good joke and I laughed. I just hung out and after a while, the 'quad' on my left introduced himself as he extended his limp hand to me. For a second, I was exhilarated to be connected with the "group," but then I felt like the elk caught in the car lights again. "How can I introduce myself if I can't speak . . . I'll be embarrassed . . . how can I shake hands when I've barely used this limb. But wait . . . he's using an 'abnormal' handshake and he's not embarrassed . . . he's really up front . . . if he can do it, I can, too! I think this is something important to remember." I looked him in the eye; he locked into my glance and I looked back at my semiflaccid, hanging hand and demanded that it move.

I visualized all the muscles doing what they were supposed to do. In my mind, it all happened perfectly, but the reality was that in order to perform the handshaking task, I had to use my shoulder's large muscles to lift my hand and the left side of my body had to swing my right arm and hand to extend my hand and connect with the other disabled young man. I got a lump in my throat due to embarrassment and blurted out, "Rod!" We looked at each other and smiled. I felt great at having accomplished more. I was noticing that the fifteen to twenty other "crips" were scoping me out and without anyone having said anything, I could tell that they were accepting and applauding as I entered and became baptized into the world of the disabled.

The atmosphere changed in the room; now everyone started jabbering and some people wheeled over and, in acknowledgment of my presence, introduced themselves to me. Up until now, I had felt that

I was totally alone on an island; but now, for the first time in a month, I felt recognized and "real," even though all my pieces didn't work (yet). But after a while, I quickly became tired. I waved to the guys and wheeled and bounced off the hall to get to my room.

I locked the wheels and parked my wheelchair next to the bed, hopped on one foot to gain access to the bathroom, and hopped back to and onto the bed. As I was staring at the ceiling and consciously watching my right eye "floating," I thought of all I'd experienced that day. It was overwhelming. I felt that I was just following the lead of others, but it still was okay. I guessed this was just the beginning of my new, uncharted future. The day was scary though exciting in some ways, especially when I accomplished the unexpected tasks. Then I quickly faded. I had a strange dream: in it, I was agile and didn't need the damned wheelchair and spoke on a par with Rhodes Scholars. Wishful thinking?

I was awakened abruptly, but still softly, by a nurse: "You're going to get an alarm clock. I'm sure that you are a nice person, but I'll only wake my husband! You're an adult and you have to be responsible for everything here. . . . " As I became conscious, my response was, "Huh, where am I and who is this white tornado that screeches?" I started wiping the cobwebs out of my fuzzy gray matter; then I remembered that I was informed during the orientation that I was supposed to get up to be ready for the daily curriculum by 8:00. "This is just like going back to school."

One of the nurses hurried me to the place of my first activity. I saw a circle of seven or eight of the buddies that I had met the night before during dinner and social period. We all nodded and said hello. I was introduced to the instructor. She was so high energy—so chirpy and bubbly—that my thought was, "Is she for real?" I tried to introduce myself and blurted out, "Rod!", while pointing to myself. She extended her hand, pulling me into the group. She began explaining about this "Physical Therapy: Gross Motor Exercise" class. She went on, "You aren't competitive with each other but with yourself. You're supporters and motivators for each other and you're here to develop strong camaraderie." She started doing exercises and giving commands, "Right hand up, up to the sky! . . . arms down slowly . . . let them down . . . next to your side . . . now, shake them loose! . . . okay, extend them out to your side!"

I was trying to follow directions, keep up, and look at the instructor so I could understand the task. At the same time, I had to stare and command my nonworking arm/hand/fingers so I could fulfill the tasks. Before I began doing the exercises, I thought, "This stuff is so easy, a baby can do it!" When I started exercising, though, I realized that those thoughts were coming from my prestroke mind-set. Exercising was another humbling experience. I kept staring angrily at the part of my body that was being exercised. Sometimes certain muscles didn't respond at all; some would just twitch or make a small motion, but some reacted pretty well. By the end of the fifty-minute session, I was not only worn out; I was excited because I noticed that some muscles had reacted better than I'd expected.

During the session, I noticed that some of the others were able to do more than I and others not as much. I knew I wasn't supposed to be competitive, but I needed to check with the other guys so I could have a point of reference as to where I was within this microworld and use it to gauge how much I had to do to get it together enough to reenter the outside world. My reaction was, "I'm really screwed up! and, "Boy, do I have a long way to go!"

Everyone started rolling away from the group, and I guessed it was time to do the next thing—whatever that was. Just as I was beginning to wonder where I was supposed to go, a woman approached me. "Are you Rod?" "Uhhuh," I said, as I nodded. "You're supposed to be with me for an hour. I'm your physical therapist. My name is Terri. This is my office," she said as she wheeled me into a cubicle containing a chair and an exercise table. She reviewed my information sheet on the clipboard. I couldn't help but wonder what was on the sheet. Terri finally said, "Let's get you up on the table and we'll see what we can do." She wanted me to get from my wheelchair onto the table under my own steam as much as possible so that she could assess what type of work and how much of it "we" would have to do. The goal was for me to learn some techniques for mobility and physical exercises to retrack muscle strengths and coordination. She waited while I tried to think through what I had to do to get up out of the wheelchair and onto that table.

Terri noticed my apprehensiveness; she put a hand on my shoulder and expressed a desire to help me. "I think I can show you some easier and more secure ways to move around." I turned my head around to question her statement's validity and almost lost my balance until she put her other hand around my waist and placed one of her legs against my ineffective thigh. I looked into her eyes and saw steadiness, compassion, and a sparkle of excitement; with that acknowledgment, she helped me up onto the table. She gave me an excellent back massage and then showed me stretch exercises to do with my right limbs so that she could see what she had to work with. She raised, pulled, twisted, pushed, grabbed, tugged, bent, rotated, turned, curled, and contorted all the muscles in my limbs. I was watching it all, but I still wasn't actually "feeling" what I should be feeling!

When she completed that testing, she said, "Now I want to see how much you can do by yourself. I'll tell you what to move and you do your best. Raise your leg as far as you can." I was lying on my back. I tried like hell to raise that listless leg; it trembled a bit and finally rose about two inches off the table. Then she told me to move my arm, foot, hand, fingers, toes, knee, elbow, and a couple of other parts. Then we went through it again. I was getting angry because the muscles were either not doing anything or barely doing what they were supposed to. I kept looking at the specific area where something more should have been happening. "I know they can do it! How can I figure out how they are supposed to look or feel? The muscles on the left side can do it; why not the right side? How can I teach these flaccid muscles to function again? If my brain tells the left leg to lift, how does that feel? I'll try this . . . " I stared at my left leg and gave the command. "That was so fast! Now I'll try to really slow it down."

I tried to visualize how the command went from each synapse to the next until it got back to the destination and then saw it translate from command into action. I saw it go from my brain to the leg, and then the leg began to respond. "Okay, now I see how that one works; can I do the same thing with the right leg?" I stopped for a moment, closed my eyes, and formed a crystal-clear image of what should happen. As I kept that image, I opened my eyes, commanded the task, and watched the results traveling through my muscle system to the target. The leg slowly rose further than it ever had before—about a foot.

"My God! It can be done! This is how to do it! I found the key!" I grinned at Terri like a Cheshire cat, and she smiled as she shared in the excitement. "Wow! This . . . leg . . . how . . . done . . . wow! . . . saw . . . it! . . . wow!" I recognized that this was just the beginning and that I would have to work on it a million more times to get anything together, but right then, my miracle began to unfold! I stopped for a moment, conjured up the image and everything else to do in the same sequence, and got ready to increase the intensity of my actions. Then I pushed the "go" button. "It worked again! Okay, Rod, let's try all the other muscles that have to be fixed!" I tried to do as much as I could right then; during that experience of exercising the arm and everything else, I lost myself in my enthusiasm. I didn't realize that my clothes were soaking wet due to the fact that I was sweating profusely. I also didn't realize that I was worn out until I fell off the table and Terri caught me and helped me get back into the wheelchair. She stated that our session was over and that it was time for lunch. "Rod, you are doing great! You don't always have to work quite as hard as you did today, though. I'm glad to know you and I'll see you at the same time tomorrow."

When therapy was finished for the day, I wasn't sure if there were further activities. As I was wheeling back to my room, I passed the exercise room. I stopped and thought of checking out all the equipment; my eyes gazed across the fifteen-foot-square, raised exercise mat, wall weights, several different sizes of sandbags, futon mats in all shapes and sizes, some free weights, and stationary bicycles. At the end of my scanning process, I saw a stand-up, wall-sized mirror at the end of a thirty-foot-long padded walkway with grab bars constructed especially to be used to practice walking. "I guess that's to help me learn to walk. How can I do that?" I tried to visualize how I could transfer from the chair to the left grabber. "That looks so precarious that I can't quite crystallize the image right now . . . soon, though!"

A couple of my peers were wheeling past me and commenting, "Hey, Rod! It's dinnertime; let's chow down!" My imagery was distracted by the calls from my new buddies and my stomach; I returned the calls with gurgles as if announcing, "I'm coming *right now!*" I slowly pointed my wheelchair toward the multiactivity room and hurried to catch up with the guys and consume massive quantities of food. In actuality, it was still an extremely complex task to wheel from point A to point B. As I arrived and positioned myself at the dinner table, I remembered that everything was more intricate and more difficult now.

I looked around and saw the guys and the nurses. Again, I realized that going through the eating chore wouldn't be easy. I looked for the nurse who had helped me so much the night before but couldn't find her. "How can I do this without her?" I shivered for a second, but I knew I could do it by myself. Dinner was a hamburger and fries, and the task turned out not to be too difficult. However, I missed my mouth a lot so I did get messy with drippings of grease, ketchup, and mustard all over me. Also, I knocked my milk over because I had forgotten that the glass was to my right where my peripheral vision had been eliminated.

As I was eating I thought I was doing okay, but when I finished, I looked at my hands as well as at the area surrounding my dinner plate and thought, "What a mess!" And as I meekly glanced around to see if anyone had noticed that I had made a mess and to see if there was a staff member to assist me, I noticed a large mirror on the wall. As my eyes went past the mirror, I looked back, paused for a moment—that was actually me in the mirror! "Oh my God!" My soul shuddered at the reality of what I saw. The "a picture is worth a thousand words" saying flashed through my mind. I felt devastated first because I saw a severely "handicapped" young man, rather than the vibrant, robust adult who had previously been invincible; second, there in the mirror was an adult-sized baby that couldn't eat without putting more food around him than into his mouth! Temporarily, I felt as if my motion got knocked off track and I had to grasp at the edge so that I wouldn't slip and fall down into the abyss, swirl down to the bottom of depression, and wallow in self-pity until I felt as though I would drown in it.

My eyes swelled, my throat clenched, and my psyche grasped for survival tools so that I might set my sights on the future and go forward, no matter what. "I've got it!" I knew at that moment that I must never give up, even when confronted with seemingly overwhelming situations. I looked at my other side—at least I was trying. It was better than it had been a little while before! After a while, a nurse came over to help me clean up the mess. I appreciated her help, but at the same time, I was angry because her actions signaled an acknowledgment of my situation. I was also embarrassed—as if I were a two-year-old kid caught doing something I shouldn't have and didn't know how to fix it. She finished her task. Generally, everyone started settling down and began conversing. Hanging out with the guys after dinner provided a great feeling. It was even better that night because it felt as if I had graduated from my "rookie" status.

I looked up at the wall clock. It was almost 7:00; I anticipated some visitors and had heard some familiar voices down the hall. "Bye, guys" went through my mind as I nodded and smiled while I tried to wheel toward my visitors so that I might socialize with them. It was my parents and two of my brothers. I tried to show them the different exercise rooms in the activity center and attempted to explain what I had learned and accomplished in just the first day. I garbled my words; my snail-paced attempts to say simple words got quicker as a result of realizing that I could then do some things I couldn't have done two days earlier. We went to my room and talked for a while. They left when I started to fall asleep. During the days I spent there, I so anticipated the evening visits from my family and friends—all the time wishing that they would never have to leave once there. That feeling reminded me of a baby or toddler just wanting its parents to always be nearby.

About the eighth evening of hanging out with the guys in the multipurpose room, I was at one of the circular tables mostly listening; whatever the subject being discussed was, I nodded and acknowledged that I was listening and understanding. Two of the six people were playing chess. After a while, I was distracted from the conversation by the men playing chess. While I was watching the game, my thoughts surfaced and I said to myself, "You know, I used to be pretty good at this game. My father taught me well and I've beaten practically everyone since I was six years old. I would really like to play again, but I don't know . . . I doubt if I would be any good. I mean, the logic and thinking process in my mind is all boggled up; whenever I try to think of a specific subject, it's lost or fragmented. My efforts to think in a sequential process or to make multioptional plans in response to change are far from being up to par."

While I was thinking these negative thoughts and following each chess move to completion, I heard, "Hey, Rod! Do you want to play the next game?" "Huh? . . . Yeah, ah, . . . used to . . . a . . . good, game, yeah!" We set up the chessboard. My mind was racing, "What am I getting into? The guy I was about to play had been beating everyone so far; he'll blow me out of the water . . . Rod! you're going to do it! Concentrate! Check your memory banks. You *can* do this. We'll see how it goes. You have nothing to lose and everything to gain . . . " My palms were getting sweaty. I felt my body getting jittery and I actually felt my brain cells popping. That part of my gray matter hadn't been tapped for quite a while. It was like turning on the ignition key of an old Chrysler with a big, eight-cylinder hemi-engine. It cranked over a couple of times; you could feel that the strong battery was strained, trying to turn over all that weight and resistance. You could hear a couple of spark plugs' electrical snaps while the rest of the cylinders became aligned. All of them were strongly running in synch, as it slammed into gear, pulled to full speed, roaring and revving as it went. "We are ready for a real game!" And my sense of competitiveness and aggressiveness became my mind-set (even though in the back of my brain, I was scared to death!). I picked up the white pawn and started slowly. The game evolved and undulated; after I got a handle on it and got into the groove, it became ferocious! It was push and pull. I was definitely sweating. I was focused. I totally forgot I was handicapped! I grinned. I looked at my competitor. I then moved the queen and actually shrieked, "Checkmate!"

Another important experience occurred during the third week of this second hospital stint. So much was happening; I'd actually begun to walk (rather than hop); I was eating with my right hand, beginning to communicate again, feeling that I was worth something through developing friendships with other patients . . . It seemed as if things were starting to roll in my direction. On this particular day, as soon as I got out of the last class, a bunch of friends showed up and all of a sudden we were having what resembled a party—just like the old days!

After a couple of hours of excitement, everyone filtered away but left such a great feeling behind. Within five minutes after the last friend left the party, my family members started filing in! Even though the hospital was twenty-plus miles away from Tacoma—where my family, my closest friends, and my fiancée were located—someone would always visit every afternoon and practically every night. From the first wave of exhilaration, and even before I had a moment of relaxation, I was excited at receiving so much attention! It was another wonderful couple of hours socializing with some of my closest people! I was so excited that I even started to forget where I was and why I was here! When everyone had to eventually leave, I was nothing but a smile. Everyone was finally gone; I realized I hadn't eaten dinner yet. In actuality, I was still so exuberant that I really wasn't very hungry, but I wheeled to the multipurpose activity room to grab something to munch on. As I was chewing on some leftovers, I realized what was missing in the midst of all the excitement. At that moment, Linda's arms came from behind me. She embraced and then kissed me. "Yeah, that's what I was missing!"

I instantly became as exhilarated as I was earlier in the day; the feelings were at least as great but more channeled since it was a one-on-one focus. We spoke (most of it was her expounding and me nodding) for a while, catching up since the last time she had visited (the day before). While she took a breath, I tried to explain how much I had accomplished in just the short period of time since she was last here. I was too excited and my language got all mixed up. While I was trying, I noticed in her eyes that nothing was making any sense to her. Therefore, I tried harder and harder. My anxiety increased; the more I tried, the more I got bogged down and the angrier I became. It was like being stuck in quicksand. The more I tried to get out of it, the worse it got.

As soon as I was totally stuck, I started fuming and blaming it on her. She at least attempted to understand my garbled words. She also really attempted with compassion to grasp my experience. She hugged me tightly to get rid of my anger, frustration, and insecurity. After a moment, she did soothe my ruffled feathers. She settled me down so I could think, "Okay, if I can't say it, I'll show her!" I took her hand and wheeled to the exercise room. I tried to point out my physical triumphs of the last few days. She acknowledged it all by becoming closer and warmer. Then she wheeled me to my dorm and helped me transfer from the chair onto the bed. We lay together for about an hour, feeling the past and denying the pain of the present. Just embracing made me feel like I was a man without problems. Both of us enjoyed the closeness, but just as we were falling asleep, the nurse doing the rounds switched the bright room light on. Linda had to go soon anyhow. It took me another fifteen minutes to go thirty feet from the room to the elevator and finally say "bye."

When the elevator doors closed, I wheeled away and shifted to a comfortable chair. I reviewed this exciting day: the parties, friends, family, conversations, jokes, caring, stories, Linda, feelings, closeness, bonding, my surviving, people's support, priorities, folks, and family. Soothed by my thoughts of these wonderful people in my life, I suddenly shivered; my palms became clammy and my forehead broke out in a sweat. I was in shock! I got a sudden jolt of reality! Even though I may have the absolute best of everything—parents, family, friends, services (I mean everything)—*it is still all up to me!* My life is my responsibility. Support and services are great, and I don't know what I would do without them, but it all comes back to me. Right then, I felt as if I was naked to the elements of the Antarctic! I continued shaking. "What am I going to do? I couldn't handle the world very well so far; how could I do it now?" Even though I was exhausted, I remained tense through the night, until I saw the sun come up.

6

Who Am I
Now?

As we have just seen in the poststroke life of Rod McLean, individuals often experience a change in identity while adapting to a stroke. Major transformations frequently occur in the way they appear to other people as well as in the way they appear to themselves. Some stroke survivors perceive themselves as being the same person, but like Rod, they must confront the fact that they now have a body that does not function as it used to and as they would like it to.

Georgia explained that she felt quite alienated from her body when she first confronted her poststroke condition: "I 'hated' the fact that I was paralyzed and still am. I felt like a stranger to myself. I had to learn how to function in this new body. I had to learn how to be this new person. It was so strange to me. I didn't like the new Georgia." She went on to note that "it took me quite a while to adjust to a body that wouldn't do what I wanted it to do. And a mind that didn't think or remember the things I used to. I felt so bad about it, but I couldn't let this stroke get the best of me, so I had to get strong and face each day with courage. I felt like a child with a new toy. My toy was the new me." She later declared that "I have learned to live with the fact that this stroke has changed me physically and mentally. But the 'old Georgia'—who is inside me—still can love and care just like she used to and that will never change." For Georgia, the outer reality that other people see may have changed, yet she is still the same person inside and still can do those things that are most important in her life—loving and caring.

Other stroke survivors do not as easily adapt to these new realities. This is particularly the case among those who are highly influenced by the impressions that others have of them (or that they suspect others have of them). These survivors are inclined to perceive themselves as being new, unacceptable people or as being "nonpeople" who must somehow establish a new identity as a result of the profound impact of the stroke on their appearance and functioning.

Sheila's first impression of her new body were very traumatic. On one occasion, soon after her stroke, her son found her naked, standing in front of her mirror crying and wondering how anyone could ever love her the way she was. She viewed herself as a new person who was much less attractive than the old Sheila. Beth observed that she now exercises in bed every morning before taking a two-mile walk. However, she sadly noted that this is just to keep her present level of movement and that no matter what she does, she will not get any better. Beth was tearful and her voice lowered as she looked at her left hand and stated, "It will never go away." As a result of her disability, she has lost her role as the host of large family gatherings during the holidays and in shopping for and wrapping Christmas presents. She also spoke of losing a certain sense of being carefree, because she now has to think about keeping her balance "every minute" and fears every time she gets on the bus that it will jolt and she will fall down. Beth also talks about missing the ability to hold her young grandchildren.

Coming to Grips with Poststroke Conditions

When people first confront the fact that they have had a stroke, it is often most helpful for them to receive some words of encouragement and for them to believe that they can overcome the physical limitations imposed by the stroke. Yet, at some point, these stroke survivors must confront the fact that some things are permanently changed in their lives. In some sense, they are different people now and must begin the process of change. Their old home—their physical and psychological sense of self—has been destroyed or is at least in disrepair. They must begin the process of reconstructing themselves and their lives.

In confronting this fact, they typically must move through a period of grieving for the loss of their old self. Survivors such as Eldon miss their favorite hobby—in his case, reading. Many more men, like Todd, primarily miss their role as a breadwinner and professional. Todd had been a high school science and physical education teacher. It was particularly difficult for him to accept the fact that he could no longer read—a core element of his professional identity—and had to quit teaching school. He became tearful when talking about the students that he no longer sees. He was unable to proceed with the interview because of the grief and pain associated with this realization. For many of the men we interviewed, work is a central part of their identity, whether this be a paying job or a postretirement hobby or recreational activity. Similarly, work inside or outside the home is often central to women's identity. Whereas the men have often retired from their jobs, the women we interviewed (coming from a more traditional era) are likely to still be active in taking care of the home and in performing various community, church, or social functions. A stroke can severely disrupt these habitual and meaningful activities.

Bob, like Todd, found that he was unable to control his emotions when it came to talking about his work-related losses. Following his stroke, Bob feared that his life, which had been based on his profession, would fall apart and that he would never be able to return to work and support his family. He felt sorry for himself and was discouraged and hopeless. He didn't know where to go for help and wasn't accustomed to dealing with his feelings. He felt he was "horrible to be around" and was burdensome to his family, who tried to be supportive. Bob admits that he wasn't in touch with what he needed from his family, so he couldn't ask for help. He still experienced a great deal of guilt about how he treated his family following the stroke.

Another survivor, Jose, was an accomplished painter who had worked for over thirty years in the field. He was still working when he had his stroke. Afterward, he became slightly aphasic and found it too difficult to go back to his office and communicate with his co-workers. He also became quite emotional and would cry when he realized his losses. He was embarrassed when he cried at the office in front of peers. Jose spent several months at a rehabilitation center, working with speech, occupational, and physical therapists. He realized that he could not go back to his old peer group and feel comfortable again. He then decided to find a new group. He joined a stroke support group, which was made available to all clients who are in therapy or to other people in the community who have experienced strokes. He found that this group helped him rebuild his self-esteem and sense of self-worth. He has become a recognized leader in the group and a motivating force and example for new members. Jose was honored with an award for service during Stroke Month in May 1992.

The women we interviewed—with or without careers—also found the limitations imposed by their stroke difficult to cope with. They could no longer operate as they used to in their professions, in their role as the pillar of their family, or in their role as breadwinner. Roberta had studied dance and music since she was fourteen years old and had hoped to become a professional singer. While this dream was never realized, she had continued to identify herself with her vocal capacity. Now, almost forty years since she first formulated her adolescent dreams, she can barely speak and must work regularly with a speech therapist to recover the skill that was the core of her identity for so many years.

Roberta also lost the use of her right arm. As a result, she had to learn to do things with her left hand. She reflected on the fact that as a young person she had been left-handed, but her parents considered left-handedness a handicap and discouraged it. She had learned to be right-handed as a child; then, at the age of fifty-two, she needed to relearn how to write with her left hand. Thus, for Roberta there was an ironic shift back to an early identity as a "lefty" as a result of having a stroke.

If stroke survivors can no longer play golf or walk down to the corner store for a morning newspaper, then, in some basic way, their identity as competent and independent adults is threatened. The recognition of these limitations and the sense of loss can be overwhelming. The task facing stroke survivors is twofold: to recognize and accept the new realities and to somehow overcome or reframe them so that they are not so overwhelming. We offer several examples of both successful and unsuccessful attempts to cope with the new realities as a means of shedding more light on how survivors adapt psychologically.

Accepting the New Realities

Alice spent a total of seventy-four days in the hospital. She then went to a rehabilitation center, where she stayed for seven weeks. There she received speech therapy, physical therapy, and occupational therapy. She doesn't remember much about the time she spent in the hospital or in the rehab center. Somewhere near the end of her stay in the rehab center, however, she recalls finally coming to the realization that things had changed dramatically in her life. Her doctor had told her that she would never walk again. At this juncture, she had the choice of giving up or moving forward with her rehabilitation. Alice remembers saying to herself: "Well, what can I do to get better?" She then began working very hard at her therapy and improved rapidly, exceeding her doctor's predictions. Another stroke survivor—Georgia—put it this way: "Somehow stroke [survivors] . . . have to find a way to 'cope' with their 'new life.' It's either you cope or you shrivel up and die and I wasn't ready to die."

Denial seems to be playing an important role in Alice's rehabilitation. She claimed that she was going to her speech therapist primarily to help her with her foreign accent—yet, in fact (according to her husband) the therapist is helping her recover her loss of speech after her stroke. Alice has an extremely positive attitude and a great deal of determination. Her interviewer was surprised that she minimized her weaknesses (such as speaking problems) and focused instead on how to get better. She mentioned several times that she had "beat" her doctor's predictions about the outcome of her disabilities. She said that she never got depressed or down about having a stroke. "Why get that way when you can do something about it?"

When asked what her impressions were of her "new body"—a body that couldn't do things that it could do before—Alice replied, "It's a nuisance. I hope it goes away. I'm doing exercises and I'm slowly improving." She said that it is frustrating that she can't do some things. She stopped driving after the stroke because she realized that she wasn't ready to drive, so she has to rely on her husband to drive her places. Alice also indicated, however, that she has found something that seems to work for her in helping her confront her body's limitations. When she is swimming in the pool, her left leg doesn't move like it should. Alice's doctor told her that the message was not getting through from the brain. So she started sending messages to her leg in Hungarian, which is her first language, and her leg started responding.

Whether this is another example of denial and wishful thinking or an exceptional new approach to physical therapy, Alice's strategy moves her out of the role of victim and gives her a healing sense of empowerment. She has become an active, problem-solving participant in her own therapeutic process. Such a positive, proactive stance can't help but be of real value to her new sense of self as well as her physical rehabilitation. Alice has not accepted the fact that she may have disabilities for the rest of her life. Instead, she continues to work hard in overcoming the effects of the stroke, and it seems so far to have been successful for her. She feels that if she works hard enough, she will get back to where she was before her stroke. This may not be realistic, but it might be self-fulfilling to at least some extent.

Self-fulfilling prophecies seem to be the key to a successful recovery for many stroke survivors. If they firmly believe that recovery is not only possible but highly likely, this belief in and of itself seems to increase the probability of successful recovery. The survivors will be more highly motivated, will not let minor setbacks deter their treatment program, and will take better care of themselves during the recovery process. Most important, the recovery process will itself be less stressful, thereby reducing the chances of yet another stroke and an even more difficult recovery process. Often the self-fulfilling prophecy builds on: (1) religious faith, (2) active participation in a variety of treatment programs, (3) ongoing professional advice and assistance, (4) enthusiastic support of other people, and/or (5) positive role models offered by other stroke survivors (as exhibited during stroke club meetings or through reading firsthand accounts such as we offer in this book). Those beginning their own recovery or helping others recover should employ one or more of these resources.

Tom recalled that the realization of profound change hit him when he returned home from the hospital. He confronted the fact that he could no longer work in his garden and that he would now have to depend on other people for all his needs. He felt a great deal of resentment at not being able to do what he had always done. Like Alice, he faced a decision: "I just wanted to give up." However, soon after Tom arrived home, his son also arrived home from the hospital, having been in a serious automobile accident. "My son had come out of his coma [following the car accident] and was ready to come home . . . so I just knuckled down and tried my best. It was damn hard." Thus, Tom was able to divert attention away from his own troubles to those of his son. Fearing his own dependence on others, Tom became aware that his son was also in need of assistance and committed himself to be there for him. He came to terms with the new reality not only of his ailing son, but also of his own limitations. During his interview, Tom often said, "Oh well, this is all I've got. I might as well live with it." His active life-style prior to the stroke has drastically changed. He now attends to his son's needs and lives a quieter, more reflective life.

Sheila described herself as virtually having to learn everything all over again. It was like being an infant, but much more difficult. She could not cook, bathe, apply makeup, walk, speak, read, write, or drive. Once again, a decision had to be reached. She repeatedly stated, "I just started over again. I had to or I would be crippled all my life." It became imperative that she learn these things in order to regain a sense of independence. Living with any of her children would have been possible for Sheila. However, like Tom, she feared becoming too dependent on others. Furthermore, she realized that they had their own lives to live.

Sheila has accepted her limitations but continually learns improved ways of functioning. She practices learning new words and writing every day on her own. Her approach to the "new self" is practical in that she is the same person, except at times when she is tired and her thoughts do not connect with her speech. Perhaps most important, Sheila has discovered that the skills she learned prior to the stroke can be relearned. However, if there was something (such as yard work) that she didn't do prior to the stroke, it would be extremely difficult to learn how to do it after the stroke. There are some things she did not like to do before the stroke. However, if she does them now, she will learn new things. For example, she now watches television because she has become primarily a visual and auditory learner rather than someone who "learns by doing."

After Susan realized that she was paralyzed on her right side and could not walk or talk, she immediately began working with her speech and occupational therapists to regain these functions. Although she worked diligently with the physical therapist to improve her strength and flexibility on the right side, to date she is still paralyzed. Facing this very difficult prospect of lifelong paralysis, Susan began reading all the literature she could find on strokes. By obtaining this information, she thought that she would find a cure for her condition. This belief was a coping strategy. It empowered her to become an active participant in her recovery and to retain hope under conditions that would lead many to despair.

By contrast, Jane believes that her ignorance regarding strokes and recovery from strokes has been helpful, for it has helped her minimize the pain associated with a full awareness of the implications of strokes for her own personal future. She openly admitted not asking questions of either the doctors or her family when she was at the hospital. Her stay in the hospital was brief, with some physical therapy; she has continued physical therapy on an outpatient basis.

For the past two years, she has been determined to regain her strength and previous level of functioning and appears to have been quite successful in this regard. Her self-determination, strength, and courage are admirable and relate directly to her denial and avoidance of "bad news." She feels that her stroke is part of the aging process and that at her age, "something is bound to go wrong." It appears that despite her denial, she has been able to accept the stroke and has been active in her own rehabilitation. Thus, while Susan has used knowledge about strokes as a central ingredient in her self-directed rehabilitation, Jane has been able to engage actively in her own rehabilitation precisely because she can live with the fiction that her stroke was simply part of the normal aging process and that she can successfully cope with this "aging issue," as do many other men and women as they grow older.

Margaret, like Susan, has effectively faced her stroke-related limitations by becoming knowledgeable about strokes and by taking an active role in her own therapy. Unlike Susan, however, Margaret has focused not so much on recovery from the stroke she just had but rather on avoiding the occurrence of another stroke. She blames herself for having had the first stroke but has directed her self-anger toward increased attention to nutrition and exercise.

Some of Margaret's anger has also been directed toward the medical profession. She does not have all that much faith in the advice of her doctors, preferring to make decisions herself. She recently "fired" her internist of many years, engaging a family practitioner who had been recommended by a friend. While the new physician may be no better than the old, Margaret at least gained the satisfaction and empowerment associated with choosing her own doctor. She has done an effective job of converting anger into action. She didn't so much want to blame herself or her doctor for her difficulties as she wanted to assume control for her own rehabilitation. She wanted to know who was responsible for her current condition so that she would know how to conduct the rest of her life: "My doctor should have been more clear . . . my husband is responsible for this . . . I am responsible for that."

Another successful strategy for Margaret is what her interviewer described as "healthy resignation" to the fact that she will never quite be who she was before the stroke. Like Rod and many of the other stroke survivors we interviewed, Margaret faced an early choice and could have easily given up: "At first, when I couldn't even talk, I wished God had taken me. I felt old and useless." However, like Rod and Sheila, she recognized that she could be effective in relearning how to do things she was accustomed to doing before her stroke: "I do things so much slower, but I can still take care of [my husband] and my home . . . nothing has really changed." By the end of the interview with Margaret, it became clear that it was supremely important for her to be able to take care of her husband and her home just as she had before the stroke. Like Tom—who attended to his son's rehabilitation from a car accident—she was able to shift her attention from her own troubles to the care and feeding of her husband and home. In her case, however, this "care and feeding" affirmed that "nothing has changed," whereas for Tom, this was a new poststroke condition.

Margaret was proud of the fact that she has learned to sew again and likes to practice by darning socks: "I don't care if no one else does it any more. I still think it is silly to throw out a good pair of socks just because they get a hole in the heel!" Margaret's continuing efforts to return to established, prestroke practices were particularly impressive because her physical movements have been significantly impaired by the stroke. Her right arm and hand were not only weakened by the stroke but were left in a state of constant spastic contraction. She indicated that she was still improving and that the physical therapist told her she might get back much more use of her hand and arm over time. She showed her interviewer an exercise device she uses to improve the strength of her hand.

The discrepancy between the extent of Margaret's actual disability and her perceived disability was impressive and demonstrated the important use of denial in the healing process. Perhaps she will never be able to do what she used to do in her home and with her husband. Perhaps she really isn't taking very good care of either her husband or home. Her husband might be assuming increasing responsibility while being careful not to shatter his wife's illusions that "nothing has changed." Would it be better to confront Margaret with the "reality" of her condition? Probably not. Once again, her wishful thinking may be self-fulfilling: she may be getting better, despite the doctor's prognosis, precisely because she thinks she *will* get better.

Like Margaret, Greta does a good job of mixing denial and wishful thinking with active involvement in her own recovery. She contended that not knowing what the future will hold can sometimes be helpful. "In the beginning," she said, "if anybody had told me [that the length of my rehabilitation] would have been three years, I don't know how I would have been able to cope with it." She indicated, however, that the three years have "gone by very fast." She thinks the secret is to work very hard and to "always think good thoughts and positive thoughts." She works very hard indeed. She rises at 6:30 each morning to do exercises with a program on public television. She also has an exercycle, which she rides faithfully for fifteen to twenty minutes several times a day. During her interview, Greta was always in motion, constantly exercising her arm or moving her leg. She has engaged in massage therapy, water therapy, physical therapy, and constant exercise to overcome her disability. She still wears a brace on her leg to keep it from "drooping" but said she was once told she'd always walk with a cane. "*Always* and *forever*," she declared, "are words that just aren't in my vocabulary."

Betsy offered us another example of successful acceptance of the new reality associated with recovery from strokes. In her case, however, recovery was made more complex as a result of a second major intrusion in her life—the death of her husband. Betsy felt that her identity has not changed much as a result of the stroke. She said it was hard, but she was able to accept that she couldn't go back to work and applied for disability retirement. Her husband died at work of a heart attack three years after she had her stroke. Betsy repeatedly mentioned that the impact of her stroke really hit her only after the death of her husband. She still worries that his death may have been related to the additional stress associated with his caring for her after the stroke. She felt even more grief after her husband's death than she did after having the stroke and would often wake up crying at night when she still lived in the home they had shared. Betsy missed him most at night and was faced more directly with having to do things for herself after his death. She moved about a year later to a flat in a building owned by one of her children. Family members now live above and below her. She still experiences occasional sadness and anger when she can't do things that she could do before the stroke but, on the whole, is coping well.

The key to Betsy's successful recovery from her stroke seems to be the supportive family environment in which she finds herself—perhaps in part as a result of the death of her husband. She has begun to assume the role that her own grandmother played in living with Betsy and her husband prior to Betsy's stroke. Her grandmother apparently always kept the address book with everyone's whereabouts, and family members would call her to connect with each other. Betsy began to assume a similar role as head of the family. This accelerated after her stroke and her grandmother's death. During her interview, Betsy received several phone calls from family members and was in the process of caring for her grandchildren and helping make arrangements for them for the evening. Like Tom (in caring for his son after the auto accident) and Margaret (in apparently taking care of her husband and home), Betsy finds meaning and a role in life following her stroke by taking care of other people in her life—even though there are now physical limitations with regard to the role she can play.

Betsy did experience some tension with her youngest daughter after her stroke, when her daughter wanted to help her. Even though she didn't want help, she felt it was not polite to turn down this assistance. She eventually talked to her daughter about this dilemma and is now more straightforward with her. Like many of the people we interviewed, Betsy is trying to be as independent as possible and is actually concerned more with being able to help others than with receiving help herself. As we will see in the last section of this book, this can cause major problems for caregivers, who often are more interested in providing assistance to the stroke survivors than in receiving assistance themselves.

Like Susan, Margaret, and Greta (and most of the other successful survivors we interviewed), Betsy feels that her primary strength is her positive attitude about recovery from the stroke. It allows her to move through her difficulties and to participate in many rehabilitation activities. In addition to taking part in social groups, she goes to a local recreational facility and has joined an exercise class. She feels good about the positive feedback she has gotten from other stroke survivors when she has taught the class (the regular teacher being out with the flu). Betsy seems very proud of being able to use her positive attitude to help others as well as herself. She serves as a grandmother to people in her family and as an adviser and cheerleader to other stroke survivors. While she appreciates receiving assistance from other people—for example, when strangers help her in the grocery store when she can't reach something—she is resistant to extensive assistance, particularly from family members. Coming from a close and highly supportive family, Betsy has many role models in her life for the provision of caring services; however, she also recognizes the need for some boundaries in this highly enmeshed family. She is hesitant about receiving too much care for herself and thereby losing her hard-won courage and highly interdependent family.

In stark contrast to Betsy, Sean was living alone at the time he had his stroke, and he continues to struggle by himself with rehabilitation. When he awoke in the middle of the night following his stroke, Sean realized that he could not control his body: "I knew something was seriously wrong." He struggled to dress himself and arouse his neighbors, who called the hospital. He described being frightened but not feeling pain. He was particularly fearful about the loss of control, the potential loss of independence, and the absence of a supportive social system: "It was scary. I didn't know if others would really help me." At the time of his stroke, Sean was solidly career oriented, having obtained both master's and doctoral degrees, and took great pride in his autonomy. He informed the interviewer that his sister had brought his bills to the hospital three days after the stroke and that he personally took care of his business during this period of recovery. Sean is clearly competent and highly invested in retaining this competence.

Sean's concerns for autonomy were clearly motivators in his recovery: "I wanted to be independent. I wanted to gain everything back so I wouldn't have to rely on others." He was fortunate. He suffered decreased physical functioning on his left side but was able to regain his full range of motion with minimal loss of strength. His recovery became "an obsession." Although his brothers helped him, he immediately focused on directing and implementing his own physical recovery, seeing himself (as did many of the other successful survivors we interviewed) as primarily responsible for the actions he knew were required. He said that the physicians he worked with were very informative about his physical condition, but that "not much" psychological service had been provided.

Thus, for both Sean and Betsy, autonomy was important. They both wanted some control over the amount of assistance they received. Unlike Betsy, Sean began with minimal family support and seems to be making it pretty well on his own. He asks for little assistance, focuses primarily on his own recovery, and provides little assistance to other people. Sean is an island and needs little outside help, though one wonders what would have happened if his stroke had been more severe and if he had had to face a future that would require him to become more dependent on others.

What seem to be the key ingredients associated with successful acceptance of the limitations imposed by strokes? First, *denial* is often needed—though this denial shouldn't take the form of massive indifference to or avoidance of the realities facing the stroke survivor. Rather, denial should be built on optimism and wishful thinking: I know that I have a hard road ahead, but I choose to consider my prognosis to be positive and my path free of insurmountable barriers.

Like many of the successful survivors we interviewed, Kari established a positive life narrative for herself after her stroke. She spoke of her body as healthy and of her self as filled with hope and new life. While, on the one hand, she finds it hard to "own" the parts of her body that have been most affected by the stroke, she has been able to preserve a sense of herself as a healthy person: "Yes, I am disabled. My body appears to be in a disabled situation, but I do feel very healthy." She used to relate to her disabled arm as somehow not part of herself. Now she tries to be loving toward her arm: "I try very hard not to be upset at my arm. Because often—see what my arm's doing right now— it just holds on. Now I work with the fact that this [points to her arm] is Kari. Kari needs love [she rubs her arm] and she deserves it and gets it." When asked if she remembers a time when she became aware of the magnitude of her stroke, Kari replied: "I never have!" Perhaps by not allowing the stroke to "hit her over the head," she was able to keep trying.

The second key ingredient in the successful confrontation of stroke-related limitations is *short-term goal setting*. Denial will only get the stroke survivor so far. It must be tempered in most cases with the identification and persistent efforts toward achievement of realistic goals. A successful stroke survivor imagines full recovery from the stroke (wishful thinking), yet sets short-term realistic goals. Carla does most things with her right hand now because, though she can move her fingers and grasp things with her left hand, it is undependable. She feels most handicapped in bed because she can't turn over or get out of bed. One of her short-term goals is to be able to do these tasks. She plays the piano by ear and has been trying to do that but says it sounds bad. A short-term goal for her is to play a little better. Carla believes she will get stronger over time. Her third short-term goal is to be able to go to the bathroom alone.

Beth is similarly responding to the effects of her stroke by blending wishful thinking and short-term goal setting. She keeps herself thinking in terms of "how can I deal with it" rather than "I had a stroke." She set a short-term goal for herself in the new year to investigate a new exercise class she recently heard about. In addition, she makes gentle and loving use of denial when she uses humor in discussing and dealing with her stroke in conjunction with her family and friends. She gave the example of playing Nintendo with her grandson. He encouraged her to go faster until he asked her, "Is that your dumb hand, Grandma?"

Third, while denial and short-term goal setting are often critical to one's ability to move beyond the initial despondency associated with the stroke aftermath, they must be balanced with a *patience* that is founded, like short-term goal setting, on a realistic base. Martin indicated that the hardest lesson for him to learn after his stroke was patience. He had to accept the fact that things were going to happen more slowly than usual. He said that it was hard for him to accept that he can't work or drive and that the skills associated with these "normal" activities will return slowly if at all. Patience often is found in the setting of short-term treatment goals. It is also found in the supportive environment provided by family members and, in particular, other stroke survivors. Many of those we interviewed indicated that they became much more patient with their own recovery after seeing other survivors who had recovered many skills over time. They observed that hard work can pay off, provided that the survivors remain diligent and optimistic in their rehabilitation efforts.

A fourth key ingredient is the *proactive stance* that successful stroke survivors take with regard to their own treatment and rehabilitation. Virtually every successful stroke survivor we interviewed spoke of one or two strategies that they use to assume control of their own recovery. This strategy could involve accepting partial or total blame for having a stroke in the first place, concluding that physicians and other medical professionals cannot be fully trusted, or believing that a stroke survivor should learn as much as possible about the disability inflicted on them.

Resisting the New Realities

The stroke survivors we interviewed are probably inclined to be among those most successful in coping with the new realities of their stroke. Men and women who have not been successful typically are less inclined to agree to be interviewed or, even more basically, are likely to be isolated and unknown to the people and institutions that referred us to stroke survivors. Yet, even among those who did agree to be interviewed, we discovered several who were not doing a good job of coming to terms with the new realities. In some instances, they were starting in a very hard place, having had much more severe strokes than those who were more successful or having been forced to live in conditions of poverty, ignorance, isolation, or family dysfunction that would make life difficult for anyone—particularly for someone who is disabled.

Yet, as we showed in several of the case studies above, many people severely handicapped by strokes have made successful adjustments. Despite facing challenging conditions such as poverty, the death of a spouse, or isolation, these survivors have been able to find the internal resources to be successful. As we examine the lives of those who have not been successful, therefore, much can be learned. These men and women can teach us about the debilitating effects of hopelessness and despair, about the interplay between lack of social support and a sense of powerlessness, and, in particular, about the impact of denial when it is pervasive and indiscriminate.

Jim was tested at a local clinic after he had a stroke and was found to be experiencing some deficits in memory, impaired right-hand motor control, and loss of vocabulary as well as other speech deficits. He reported: "I didn't recognize any difficulty in talking." Yet not only does he suffer aphasia, but he also experiences confusion in calling objects what they are. He stated: "I finally realized I had problems at work in April of 1989 when it took me so long to do anything they gave me. My boss was really nice about it, but I was embarrassed. A normal five-minute job took me several hours to finish. I felt bad if they gave me an easier job." His boss sent Jim to a company physician, who sent him to a psychiatrist for evaluation. When the psychiatrist reported to the boss that Jim's verbal IQ had fallen all the way to 80, Jim realized, "I was pretty sick." He finally left work on disability—with a 40 percent penalty—in September 1990.

After going through the tests, Jim maintained a belief that "everything would come back eventually." He had already allowed his denial of any disability to affect his performance at work and was now denying the realities of his disability to the extent that he failed to recognize the need for rehabilitative therapy. When, after a couple of years, he failed to improve, Jim became frustrated. He reports no depression or suicidal impulses—"just frustration." Like most other stroke survivors, he may have lost some of his previous abilities; however, by embracing the "new" person he has become, he can begin to make use of recently acquired skills or learn to focus on the old skills he still possesses.

Jim finally decided to "continue forward." Yet, when interviewed, he was still in denial: "I don't see myself as any different than before the stroke—I don't dwell on it." He described his frustration with being unable to write a simple letter: "I tried to write my daughter a letter, and it took me all day. I can't get what I'm thinking on paper." Yet he will do nothing to ameliorate this problem. He seems to be aware of some other difficulties. He readily admitted, for example, that his memory is "not what it used to be." Consequently, he indicated that he typically makes notes on material he has to remember. He also knows that his motor functioning is somewhat compromised, although he contended that substantial improvement has taken place.

On the one hand, Jim claimed that "most people don't see [me] as different and none treat [me] any differently." Yet several minutes later, he indicated that people are more condescending than they were before the stroke. He mentioned that he still goes snow and water skiing with his buddies but that they are overprotective with him. While he expressed discomfort with this behavior, Jim insisted that he has not been treated differently since the stroke. Clearly, he holds several different and often contradictory images of himself as a poststroke survivor. He seems to be fighting against any recognition that the world has changed for him. Yet he is making several adjustments in his own behavior to accommodate these unacknowledged changes. He is aware of differences in the way other people relate to him, while failing to acknowledge the reasons why these relationships have changed. Significant improvement in Jim's poststroke physical and psychological adjustment may have to await his acknowledgment of and direct confrontation with changes in himself and his capacity to do certain things.

When asked by the interviewer what it was like in terms of reentry into the "real world" after having a stroke, Jim was perplexed, for as far as he is concerned he has never been absent from this world. Jim believed that things would return to normal as soon as he healed. Like many others who have successfully coped with their stroke, Jim said, "I never gave up. I knew I could do it." But then he said, "Even when I got frustrated, I just accepted things." The big difference between Jim and the more successful survivors is that Jim has taken very few steps to help get things back to normal, hence they remain abnormal. Furthermore, unlike the successful survivors, Jim has not acknowledged any of the realities; hence he lives with contradictions: "I never give up" and "I just accept things." He was left at the end of his interview with little to say to other survivors, other than suggesting that they remain happy regardless of what happens and that they obtain help from other people who can help them "take it [the stroke] in stride [literally]." We are left with a man who feels powerless and relies exclusively on primitive denial and a vague hope for future recovery.

Jane offered a similar portrait of ineffective adaptation. Like many of the stroke survivors, she described her stroke as "devastating" and said she still experiences great fear, especially about having another stroke. Whereas Margaret, who also fears having another stroke, took action with regard to this fear by changing her nutritional and exercise behavior, Jane talked about simply being fearful about having another stroke and about falling down and embarrassing herself. She denied having any difficulty, however, in adjusting to her stroke: "You basically revert back to the type of person you were before [the stroke]."

During her interview, Jane consistently denied anything related to being a different person since her stroke or being seen by others as being in any sense different. Like Jim, she denied that the stroke has changed her life dramatically. If anything, according to her, her stroke has encouraged her to slow down: "Perhaps it happened to slow me down and maybe so I could see the rest of my years from a different light—I don't know why it happened . . . but I view age differently—I think there was a reason for it—maybe to help other people." While this reframing of her stroke as a blessing or message to her has certainly been used as a vehicle for rehabilitation by many stroke survivors, Jane doesn't seem to make very effective use of this perspective. First, she hasn't taken many actions that would lead to a slower life pace; rather, she has gotten even more trapped in an old family role—as protector and nurturer for everyone else in her life. The stroke did not teach her to help other people; she has been doing that all her life. Thus, the frame that Jane placed on her stroke experience only perpetuated her prestroke life-style rather than changing it in any way.

Jane assigns some blame to her husband regarding difficulties she has had in adjusting to the new realities (which she does not admit have changed!): "My husband didn't do a lot for me. He encouraged me to go back to doing what I used to do. I think my children were scared I was gonna die," Jane observed, because "they had already lost a sister and a father—but they quickly saw that I was okay." We may have discovered here the source of Jane's resistance to facing changes in her own life. Clearly, her husband and children were themselves scared. They also wanted to deny the impact of the stroke, in part (at least for the children) because Jane did survive, which was not the case with their sister and father. Jane indicated throughout her interview that family support was extremely important to her and that her family was very supportive of her—and, we would suggest, perhaps also supportive of her defensive denial.

When Jane was asked what it was like stepping back into the world,

she differed from Jim in that she admitted that it was "hard." In particular, it was hard "because of the fear—fear of falling—but I forced myself to do things." She admitted that she felt frustrated with things she
couldn't do but said, "I just sort of accept it and try not to feel sorry
for myself." Thus, at times Jane can accept her limited condition—or
at least the fear associated with these limitations. She cannot readily
accept the grieving that inevitably accompanies this recognition, however. In trying not to feel sorry for herself, she is denying the most basic
and important feeling of stroke survivors. Only when survivors acknowledge the grieving can they begin the process of mourning, thereby
moving beyond this initial impasse to other stages of rehabilitation and
even rebirth.

Jane described her role in the family and with friends as "pivotal"
and indicated that this role has not changed since the stroke. She feels
that people initially approached her carefully, "but things never changed
that much." Jane later stated that "perhaps people don't see me as different because physically I don't look like I had a stroke." She cared for
her elderly mother until her death a year ago. Jane appears to be the
family "hero" who cares for people and provides nurturance—the strong
one that everyone relies on for comfort. She seemed pleased that this
has not changed and that she still has a role in the family that has
prevented any sense of her loss—any grieving. At another point in the
interview, she mentioned that she has low self-esteem and lacks self-
confidence. Perhaps she is dependent on her family for the esteem and
confidence that she does possess. They, in turn, wish to keep her in
her prestroke role and are fearful about any change in this role (as a
result of her incapacity or death).

Jane said the most important thing she did to help herself adjust
to the stroke was to participate in a stroke support group. At first glance,
this seems like a good idea: she can begin to receive support from other
people, rather than always being the nurturer herself. Yet she went on
to note that "everything is fine—I don't have great wants." One wonders
whether she will ever make use of a support group, other than to be
once again a nurturer and provider to other members of the group. On
the one hand, Jane feels that "it is up to me if I want anything." On

the other hand, she repeatedly spoke about how important it is for her to be with other people and how helpful the support group has been. She mentioned episodes of depression before and after the stroke, yet suggested that "everyone gets depressed now and then." A breakthrough will only occur for Jane when she can begin to rely on other people for help and when she can allow herself to grieve rather than being distracted by the apparent needs of the other people with whom she surrounds herself.

Grace, like Jane, lives in a world filled with the ghosts of past deaths and old family roles and patterns. Her father had a stroke many years ago and remained in a coma for six weeks before dying. This experience made the stroke particularly traumatic for Grace. During the interview, she offered no insights into how the stroke had changed her as a person. The things she said about herself suggest that she feels she is now less valuable as a person than she was before the stroke. She is modest and unassuming and expressed appreciation of her new husband (whom she married several years ago); she said he has never uttered a bad thing about her limitations. But she feels that she does not function adequately and that her husband is being kind in staying with her. She even implied that if she had known she was going to have a stroke within a few years of their marriage, she would not have gotten married because it was unfair to him.

On the one hand, Grace said she "pushes" herself. She goes out with friends and is particularly fond of those friends she has made since her stroke who are members of her stroke group. She also takes the bus to walk in the mall each day and keeps busy by reading. She does not feel it is okay to "feel sorry for myself," but her interviewer had the impression that when she does focus on the stroke, she feels more of the loss and sadness and that is unpleasant for her. Grace indicated that people do not treat her differently, but she said several times that she is "embarrassed" by her body in public because of its limitations. Like Jane, she fears falling, as well as uncontrollable choking and vomiting. She is uncomfortable with her body even when she is alone at home. One time, she fell out of her wheelchair while at home alone and said she still felt "embarrassed."

Clearly, the issue of body image for Grace is crucial—perhaps in particular because she has recently married. While most of the people we interviewed were concerned with their body image and how other people react to their disability, they have tended to take some action and work toward the rehabilitation of their body. However, like Jane, Grace seems mostly to be bottled up with emotions—such as grief and embarrassment—that are either unacknowledged or dominate her life and limit her options (even more than her real physical disabilities do). One wonders what role Grace's new husband plays in this process of self-doubt and suppressed grief. The adjustment for him must have been difficult, and he certainly must also have to grapple with feelings of anger, grief, and embarrassment. As we will note in the final section of this book, substantial support for both stroke survivors and spouses is often critical, especially if the relationship is new and lacks the continuity and history of a long-term relationship.

Ester is yet another person who offered a story filled with hopelessness and despair. She had her stroke two years prior to the interview. She was at home when it occurred and was hospitalized at a large, nationally known hospital. She said she was extremely frightened at the time but quickly discounted these feelings, saying she was well taken care of and that her husband was helpful. She focused minimally on the pain and the actual loss of control that characterize stroke symptomology. She seemed unable to directly attend to any unpleasant or uncomfortable aspects of her personal stroke experience. Ester was remarkably uninformed about the specifics of the stroke process and resultant physical and emotional impairment. The interviewer suggested that she was passive about the world around her, was resigned to having to live with the limitations of the stroke, and used a high degree of denial, punctuated by deliberate, artificial attempts to laugh off or make light of her situation. The interviewer indicated that she felt considerable compassion, respect, and concern for Ester and other women like her.

Ester describes her life as one of isolation. She has no one. Not even her neighbors of thirty years have paid much attention or offered help after the stroke. Much as in the case of Betsy, Ester's husband died of a heart attack within a year after her stroke. But unlike Betsy, who has other family members around her, Ester has no local family. Betsy has struggled at times with too much attention from members of her family after her stroke and after her husband's death; by contrast, Ester has experienced other family members as indifferent to her fate. The interviewer noted an underlying bitterness in Ester, though she denied that she cared about the absence of any support from others. She indulged the interviewer with several stories of the callousness that other people have shown her: cab drivers who wait in their vehicles watching her descend her uneven, precarious, steep stairs alone and bus drivers impatient with her slow navigation toward a seat. Each of these seemingly small incidents served as painful reminders to Ester (and other stroke survivors) of being disabled. Frustration regarding being defined as disabled leads inevitably to anger—which is often directed against oneself rather than outward (where it belongs!).

Transportation problems and social isolation emerged as salient themes in Ester's life. What economic and interpersonal resources she had once had are now depleted and she has no way of changing this situation. Following her husband's death, she had a live-in housekeeper assist her. According to Ester, this person stole her checkbook and overdrew her account, creating extensive debts on her automatic credit card overdraft protection plan. Ester's stories were horrifying, yet she stated that her stroke "was in a place that didn't affect emotions." She denied depression, saying "it depends on where the stroke is." The interviewer commented on Ester's extensive dissociation between her emotions and the massive, negative experiences and losses that she has confronted during the past few years. Obviously, she could benefit from counseling or psychotherapy and a long-term social support structure. She is hurting and has no safe place to turn for assistance.

Some Final Lessons

The lessons that the failure experiences teach us tend to support and amplify those provided by the much more positive examples of poststroke adaptation. Clearly, denial and hope must work hand in hand with active control over one's own poststroke recovery. Denial without hope leads to despair and retreat from reality; denial and hope without active engagement in rehabilitation lead to a passive reliance on external forces and sources of authority, this often leading, in turn, to the loss of hope and to intensive despair. These negative experiences also speak to the need for a subtle balance between the old ways of doing things and the new realities. Stroke survivors do need to return to old habits and responsibilities, even if they are no longer as efficient at performing these functions. Yet stroke survivors must also be introduced to and encouraged to learn new behaviors and assume new responsibilities.

Finally, our case studies have taught us that self-esteem and a commitment to one's own recovery require that other people are thoughtful about the assistance they offer the stroke survivors. In many instances, survivors should be the ones to ask for this support rather than having to struggle with the issue of offending well-intentioned but overbearing family members or friends. Personal dignity, a sense of self-worth, and an appropriate sense of personal independence are among the most important restorative agents that stroke survivors can possess when facing the extraordinary challenge of rehabilitation.

7

Why Don't Other People Treat Me as a Person?

During the second week at the rehab hospital, the social worker approached me (Rod McLean). As she was reviewing my clipboard chart, she told me how great I was doing and suggested it would be useful for me to speak with a therapist (psychologist). "What?" I thought. "He was reviewing your case and is really excited to meet you!" she rattled on. "You're supposed to meet him over there where his office is. Okay?" She hurried away without expecting an answer. At the appointed time, I wheeled over to his office and knocked on the door. When he came to the door, he looked down at me in the wheelchair and said in a professional tone, "Hello . . . uh . . . Mr. . . . uh?" Searching his clipboard for my name, he added, "McLean? Please come in." As I was rolling in, some thoughts passed through my mind. "Is this guy for real? He's disorganized. Is this his first day or something?" I was resisting this new rehab aspect with as many reasons as I could muster. But I also remembered the gist of what the social worker had said: "The therapist is someone you can really open up with; you can express anything and everything you want to him. It can be an excellent opportunity for you to really say what you feel. It'll be your hour. He'll be your soundingboard. He might be able to really give you some viewpoints or options that you hadn't considered. And you can trust that whatever goes on behind the door is confidential."

The first thing I noticed was that he did not extend his right hand to shake hands. He introduced himself and sat down in the plush chair behind his big desk. He settled into a comfortable spot. He leaned back enough to place his elbows on the chair's arms, then pressed his fingertips against each other, placed the tops of his fingertips under his chin, and looked at me for about five minutes. I just kind of sat there waiting for him to get things going. There was so much I wanted to say about what I was feeling and experiencing. There were millions of emotional things I wanted to share and get off my chest. Also, I had a lot of questions that I hoped he could help me answer.

Finally, he opened the discussion with a generic question or two. I tried to provide answers, but my language was mixed up and my speech was so slow that it became slurred—as if it was in slow motion. Still, as soon as I opened my mouth, I wanted to unload it all. It was as if I was so overloaded that this was the first place I felt that I could've dumped it. After I'd unloaded enough to breathe, I looked into the therapist's eyes. I shivered! He wasn't listening; he wasn't even trying! As he looked down at me, I felt devastated! I had just opened up for the first time in ages, and he was looking at me as if I was just "one of those" pitiful and useless "things" that "we professionals" are forced to listen to. We don't really give a damn about their useless existence.

He lightly offered some token advice, as if he were generously tossing out a few crumbs of brilliance. I was fuming. First my brain, then the entirety of my being was seething with rage. At the same time, my language became more and more impossible. He noted in a condescending manner that, "Yes, it's all right to be angry because you're handicapped. After a couple of months or years, you'll be okay with it. Maybe you'll even get a little job and feel better about yourself. You know, some people are worse off than you, anyhow. Things'll get better than they are right now, don't worry. Is there anything else you're worried about?"

Before I even opened my mouth, he stared at the clock pointedly. "Gosh, Mr. McLean, I guess we've run out of time. It was nice to meet you. It was really a great session; I think we both learned and gained so much . . . " My rage boiled over! "You idiot! You totally missed the mark! You don't even have a clue about where I'm coming from! Or about what I need and want! The sad part is that you don't give a damn!"

I continued fuming and stomped my wheels out of there. I wheeled, banged, and crashed against the wall. My throat was clenching with hurt. I started blaming him and other external things. I felt overwhelmed by negative energy. Just before I became strangled by failure, though, I came to my senses: "It really hurts not being acknowledged as a person! But let's turn it around! Don't believe him. I'll prove him wrong! I'll use his stupidity to nurture my positive growth!" I paused for a moment and tried to think of strategies that would be powerful enough to neutralize his negative attitude. I rolled to the walking board with bars and made a furious effort to walk better to prove to myself that "he" was totally at fault. I practiced through the day's remaining classes, through dinner, through social activities, and until I couldn't see myself any more in that cynically laughing mirror.

It had been about two weeks since I'd arrived at the rehab center and had first spotted the parallel bars—used for what's known as "walking the line"—with the mirror at the end. Every time I wheeled past those bars, I wanted to practice with them so that I could actually walk again. At 3:00, the classes were done for the day. All the others wheeled off in various directions—mainly to their own rooms or the multipurpose room. I hadn't planned anything. But as I moved past the parallel bars, I wheeled over to the beginning point, locked the wheelchair's brakes, and tried to figure out how I could use this formidable-looking contraption. In five minutes, I leaned over and reached for the bar on the left. When I felt the finely sanded wood, I shuddered. "How can I do this? It looks impossible! I've been wheeling or hopping a couple of steps at a time, but never walking. Even when I've tried to hop, the nurses were surprised and said I shouldn't do it until they say I'm ready."

My poor self-esteem and apprehensiveness sneaked to the surface. I grabbed my blinders, put them on, and adjusted them so I could only go forward and break through the barriers. I wanted to be able to accomplish this task. "Okay, I'm grasping the bar as tightly as possible and leaning forward on my left leg and foot. Now I'm springing further forward and up at the same time." I started to lose my balance, so I held the bar for a second—just long enough to project my rear end backward so that I fell back into the wheelchair. "Whew!" I took a breather in order to settle down. I then visually walked through it again so I could be up on the bars and beginning my experience of walking again.

"This is so scary because it's the unknown, Rod. But it's up to me!" I visualized and walked through it again; it looked like it should work this time. I grasped the bar, leaned forward as before, and swiveled my head, butt, and torso around to the left and forward. At the same time, I flipped my left wrist up on the bar, as though I were changing from a pull-up to a push-up. "Well, I'm up here! Let's look around. I'll get my bearings and figure out what to do to make it all the way." I looked at the bar on the left and noticed that my left hand was grasping it so hard that the knuckles had turned white. "Yes, I guess I can slide my hand all the way to the mirror end." I looked down at my legs and feet. They looked awkward, since I was leaning onto my left leg and all its muscles were flexed. My right leg was positioned behind the other one, just hanging there without any weight on it.

I was obviously not relying on my legs for any balance, stability, or strength; the muscles seemed so flaccid. "Let's figure this out . . . it's a piece of cake! . . . I'll just put one leg in front of the other . . . right!", I snickered to myself. "Okay, it's kind of like in physical therapy when I raise my leg in different ways and use different muscles. I have to watch, calculate, and remember how the muscles of the left leg work for the different parts of the walking tasks, then visualize and mentally command all the muscles and tendons to be ready to take action." In my mind, I saw my commands traveling from my gray matter down to each muscle, to the hips, then to the inside, outside, and back and front of the thighs. From there, the signals would travel down both sides of the calves, with the multimuscles combining at the ankles for the muscle distribution into the foot and toes. I had to remember another special muscle cord that travels down the front of the leg and across the top of the foot to the arch, then goes across the ball of the foot and ends up at the little toe. I had to go through this whole process so I could raise and wiggle the toes to be able to step forward when walking.

"Okay, the muscles are ready. Now I have to figure out the sequence of the muscles and the amount each gets used." I looked up and forward; I saw myself in the mirror. "It's grotesque! This is my incentive to get my act together again." I took a step with my left leg; I wanted to be sure I could do it properly, so I checked the muscles needed to walk. I stopped just for a second, double-checked everything, visualized, glared at my left leg and foot, and took the first step! "Yeah! We did it!" I tried again; I noticed that I mainly raised my left foot by raising my hip. Assessing if there were any adjustments to be made, I then applied the ones necessary to each further step. That way, I was able to use more of the other muscles that should have been fully involved.

In the beginning, every step seemed like it took an hour. When my right foot took the first step, it dragged terribly. But even though it only shuffled a distance of about six inches, the movement was still miraculous; my eyes swelled. I grasped the bar as tightly as possible; my whole body was flexed. I closed my eyes for a second to find my strength, fought off the tears, and took the next step . . . and the next . . . and eventually went to the end where that damned mirror was laughing at me. "I did it! Wow! What a feeling! Let's do it again!" I paused for a moment. "How do I turn around?" I thought it out and slowly, mechanically swiveled around. When I saw my wheelchair (my hated symbol of security) so far away at the end of the walkway, I felt so insecure. It was like learning how to swim; you stop to see how far you've gone, and when you realize the water is above your head, a frantic feeling sets in. But I regained my composure, looked at the wheelchair, focused on what I had to do, and resumed walking until I got there.

Standing there for a moment, I realized that my whole body was perspiring. I looked at the clock on the wall; it was 5:30! I felt exhilarated and exhausted—and hungry. I got back into the wheelchair, spinning around and bouncing and crashing off the wall as I headed for the mess hall. "I have to hurry and eat so I can get back to the bars to practice some more. I don't want to stop until I've really gotten the hang of it." It was like being addicted; I could never get enough of it. As soon as I finished dinner, I went back. I continued practicing until 1:00 A.M., at which point I practically stumbled from fatigue. From this day on, every extra moment was committed to this task.

I don't know how many thousands, hundred of thousands, or even millions of times that I "walked" to that mirror and back. With each lap complete, I felt better, stronger, more coordinated, more empowered, and more in control of my life. For so long, I had to actually "watch" every single step I took, making sure that all the many elements were being choreographed properly. After practicing for a long time, I could concentrate and start thinking about it at a different level—all at the same time. I had experienced and achieved so much in such a short period of time. My weak brain was only running on a minimal amount of energy, and I had so much to think about to figure my options and create a plan.

Five or six days after I had initially tried to learn how to walk using the bars, I was getting in the groove of the drill. About 4:00 (an hour after the end of my classes on Friday), the physical therapist—who had been working with me every day—was leaving her office. She suddenly noticed that I was exercising and exclaimed, "Rod, what are you doing? In our sessions, we're just beginning to get you to stand up. Why didn't you tell me?" I felt as if I had been "caught with my paw in the cookie jar." She asked, "How long have you been practicing this? If I'd known, I could've helped you even more. Can I help you right now?"

With an appreciative smile, I nodded and awkwardly blurted thanks. For the next two hours, she observed, commented, complimented, modeled, offered suggestions, and described options and cues for me to remember. She physically pushed, pulled, resisted, and lifted all the big and small muscles and continuously reminded me to look at and visualize the muscles moving, flexing, and transferring the energy from one to another to demand that the system work.

I learned a lot. She offered so many techniques and so much personal support. For example, after making one observation, she suggested, "Continue walking toward the mirror, watch your walking, and tell me what's missing from your gait." I started awkwardly because I had to walk without actually seeing my feet moving, but I continued looking at myself in the mirror. I went back and forth on the twenty-foot ramp without recognizing what I was missing. After about ten minutes of guessing everything wrong, I realized that when I walked, my right arm just hung there! When I recognized this, she coached me in taking another step toward normality. Then she noticed it was already 6:00. We looked at each other and acknowledged that both of us had worked hard and that I was sweaty. She also glistened with moisture. "Rod, it was great! You're getting better pretty quickly. If you practice over the weekend, you should be ready for some new tasks to be added to your repertoire." As we parted, she gave me a light hug.

I watched her disappear as the door closed behind her. I was impressed and thought, "She didn't have to stay around and help me. She seemed to want to help; her caring heart had motivated her to stay. 'Thanks!' She made me feel I was worth it." I stood there for a while until I began to shiver from my sweaty body cooling down. After I slumped back into the waiting wheelchair, I again wheeled and bumped the wall on the way to the dinner area. "I am going to practice the whole time until she gets back." As I solidified the commitment in my brain, I asked myself, "What are those new tasks she was referring to? I wonder if I can do them . . . " I did exercise again and again and millions of times again, while I chewed on millions of thoughts, too.

I was into my third week at the rehab center, and I felt I was one of the regulars. We, all the crips, were in transition from one class to another. I was pseudo-speaking with one of my peers. We noticed a new crip wheeling toward us. Our facial and body language was completely receptive; we wanted to welcome him into his new environment and life. We all exchanged names as we scoped each other out (like dogs sniffing at each other ritually). He appeared to be in his early sixties, a bit portly, gray hair . . . everything seemed all right, so he was well accepted and mentally embraced. He and some of the others were conversing; most of the time I listened and watched (as usual!). Then he started emphasizing how depressed and self-pitying he was. He continued along the devastating spiral of demoralization and self-condemnation. He spoke of wanting to die, and images of suicide seeped out of his mouth. To me, the bile that oozed from his anger and self-blame was like the bubonic plague seeping through villages and bringing death. I wanted to help him through his funk. I wanted to show him some options and avenues of possible success. I wanted to offer understanding and compassion. But I responded to his despair with total rejection. I didn't acknowledge his hopelessness. I tried to shout, "No! . . .

no! . . . no!", then attempted to press my own iron-clad "only going forward wearing blinders and absolutely no goddamn self-pity!" attitudes down his throat. He didn't even know what hit him, as I screeched my wheels and raced off.

Looking back on that experience, I hadn't realized that the new survivor deserved to express himself about his pain. At that time, my ego was fragile and my self-image poor. I think that when he spoke of giving up and committing suicide, the idea sneaked up on me. I think way back then, it scared the hell out of me when he touched my soul with self-pity. I'll bet my psyche in its down spiral was itself approaching the idea of suicide or of giving up in other ways. This new crip's perspective caught me off guard.

About the third or fourth day at the rehab center, I was approached by the social worker, who introduced me to the clinic's head doctor. When I looked at him, I saw his glossy wing tips, his crisp white smock with his shiny name tag, his lustrous stethoscope, his striking silver hair, his piercing coalblack eyes, and the two winged pure-white angels (nurses) floating around his regal head and trumpeting his entrance. He snapped his fingers, and the head nurse who had been following him (always by two full steps) instantly sprang to his needs. She knelt, bowed, and quietly withdrew to her station. He took the clipboard with my record from her and quickly flipped through the pages; he didn't make eye contact or even look at me. Quickly, he gave an order to the nurse to start me on some medication. He held the clipboard out for a millisecond; the nurse scurried to take it and looked at him for approval. He nodded, so she took her golden stamp—which happened to be 'God's' rubber signature stamp—and efficiently imprinted his name with authority onto my papers. As he floated away, his entourage tossed scented flower blossoms in front of him.

The next morning, a nurse met with me. She explained that the purpose of the drug (Dilantin) is to reduce the possibilities of having seizures. She also said that, at that time, research suggested that 85 percent of people who have "accidents" like mine become susceptible to epileptic convulsions. She showed me the capsules—white with a red band around the center of the torpedo—and gave me a schedule to follow.

I was supposed to take the pills three times a day: morning, afternoon, and evening. She emphasized again and again that I absolutely had to take them, or else! The "else," I inferred, would be seizures—probably grand mal! And those can kill you!

For the following three years, I took those strong little pills religiously and without exceptions. They sedated, disoriented, drugged, and screwed me up. I hated every moment under the effect of those pills. When I went back to school for some more education, I tried as hard as I could to concentrate and understand what the instructors were teaching. It was so difficult to comprehend anything when I attempted to read or ask questions. It was devastating! I had to tape the lectures and later listen to them again and again. Too much of the time, after I would read a paragraph, page, or chapter, I would realize that I had forgotten it all. My communication was damaged already because of aphasia, but the drug greatly amplified all my problems. My thinking process was slowed way down. The words were all mixed up, and when I would actually find a word, it wouldn't come out of my mouth right. A lot of the time, I was misunderstood, or my communication was so slow that people would just walk away. Occasionally, I was accused of being drunk at 8:00 A.M.

I wish the doctor had properly followed up in my situation (and every other patient's, too). He could have prescribed an electroencephalogram (EEG) or a CAT scan. If he was unwilling to do that, perhaps he should have been put on a Dilantin prescription! Maybe he could have had a lithium and Valium chaser, too! I appreciate the physician's concern that I could be susceptible to seizures. However, the medical team was way off base for three main reasons. First, they overgeneralized and assumed that I was affected by epilepsy without the appropriate testing. Second, they should have followed up to determine if the medication was necessary. Third, the medical staff was particularly insensitive to the person I was at the time. I was treated as a patient rather than a distinctive person.

Throughout the three weeks of crip bootcamp, there were some bittersweet experiences. There was one constant: I wanted to be free but was afraid to be on my own. During my original tour of the center, as we went through the multipurpose activity room, I noticed how beautiful the outside world was, as seen through the picture windows in this room. Every time I subsequently went into the room, I would gaze outside, then sigh. In a few days, I started finishing my late exercises by wheeling into the room and positioning myself closest to the world outside the hospital. My nose was practically pressed against the glass! The panoramic view was of a hill's crest extending out to rolling green farming acreage. Further on, there was a small village. It didn't matter whether it was day or night; the scene was always breathtaking and inviting. So, practically every night I finished the day staring out there into the world that I wanted with all my soul, and every time I gazed out there, it intensified my commitment to be "Rod" again.

As my rehabilitation progressed, that scenic postcard was my motivator. It kept me focused on getting back to the world. Practically every time I looked out there, in the back of my head I heard the song "Freebird." Every day the song got stronger, and toward my last day at the clinic, I had developed a "comfort zone" and in fact was getting a bit cocky. On a certain late afternoon, a bunch of my family members and Linda were at the hospital a couple of hours early as usual. Everyone was smiling as much as they had been another day almost a month ago. "Does it mean it's time to get out of here? . . . Yahoo!" I was higher than a kite! "It's been so long! I'm ready to roll!" I actually blurted, "Let's go!" Everyone exploded with happiness. When the tremor of excitement settled down just about a half note, a nurse came in to say they had been glad to meet and work together with me.

Her words and gestures reminded me that the center was safe and secure, buffered from the outside world. When that thought went through me, my jaw clenched tightly and my eyes were searching for a way back to the hospital's womb. The nurse sensitively read my fears, and she reassured me by saying, "Rod, you've done well, and in actuality there's not much more we could do for you. If there was more, you'd stay longer." Her reassurance numbed me for a few minutes as we wheeled through the corridor, went down in the elevator, and transferred into a 1965 Plymouth station wagon. When I cast a glance over my shoulder at the hospital, I thought about the experience I'd just lived through. I shuddered, realizing that I had a totally uncharted voyage ahead of me.

8

Changing Relationships

Family members, friends, and strangers all tend to shift their perceptions of people who have had strokes. Stroke survivors may look, walk, or talk a little differently. They may be confined to a wheelchair or may navigate with the assistance of a cane or walker. Confusion, emotionality, and distress may also be evident in stroke survivors. Each of these conditions tends to alienate, threaten, or somehow turn away people.

The experience of being treated as something less than a whole person is difficult for virtually every stroke survivor. Often, this concern is particularly strong for people who have been in responsible and sometimes powerful positions in their prestroke lives. They need to be able to demonstrate their continuing competence and ability to influence and impress others. The person who interviewed Martin confronted a man who had been a successful physician for many years. He had to show her constantly that he had been and still was highly successful in his career. The interviewer reported that

[as Martin was showing me documents that demonstrated to me that he had been very active in a leadership role in his local community] I was thinking to myself, "was he really on the phone [when I first arrived for the interview] or was he just telling me that he was on the phone to give me a picture of himself as he was in the past—the busy, famous pediatrician?" He wanted me to know who he was before his stroke. When I finished reading his letter to [a local social activist group], he gave me a book he wrote. . . . He asked me to look at the book. I was telling myself: "Oh God, I will never come out of this house! What is he going to give me next? Maybe it is not right to talk about his stroke? Maybe he wants me to see him as he was before the stroke and just forget about asking about his present life." I was asking myself all of these questions and at the same time I was reading the topics of the articles in the book [that Martin had handed me].

Repeatedly throughout the interview, Martin showed his perplexed interviewer the books that he had written, his picture from lectures he had given while actively involved in the local social action group, and documents from a political campaign in which he had participated. He managed to provide the interviewer with his whole biography: "family pictures . . . all I could see and know about his life." Gradually, the interviewer came to relax and enjoy the meeting with Martin. She was no longer in a hurry to start the more formal part of the interview. Just when she was losing hope of starting the interview, Martin asked, "Do you want to start the interview?" She said, "Sure, but there's no rush. I'm enjoying reading your books and knowing about you." Martin, in turn, said, "You know, after a stroke we get lonesome and if it is up to me I will keep you all day." She told him she was in no rush and would be with him as long as he wanted.

The interviewer went on to speak about Martin's vulnerability. He depends heavily on other people to buttress his own fragile self-esteem, despite a lifelong record of exceptional accomplishments. He can't do the things that he once could do and fears that people will treat him differently. He is concerned, in particular, that they will no longer be impressed by him. Some people are solicitous with Martin. Others want to help. In either case, they risk offending him because they are not showing him respect. In his rough, demanding search for attention, he will also scare away some people. He is frightened and alone. An interviewer—or colleague, friend, or even family member—who gives him "the time of day" by listening to all of his stories and expressing appreciation for his many accomplishments provides invaluable assistance. Martin and many other career-oriented people need this kind of assistance much more than they need someone who is smothering them with overprotection and condescension.

In contrast to most of the other stroke survivors we interviewed, Georgia said she really doesn't feel that anybody she personally knows treats her differently than before she had her stroke: "People treat me with the same friendliness as before." She went on to note that "one thing has changed . . . I feel people respect the fact that I didn't just give up because of my stroke." Perhaps as a result of this support and continuity of relationships, Georgia feels that she doesn't "get treated like a child at all." She notes that "I have had to learn how to use one arm and one leg. I dress myself, feed myself, and bathe myself. It's hard, but I do it. I want to walk so terribly bad, I can taste it. I am going to walk soon. I just know it and that will be the most glorious day to look forward to."

Obviously, Georgia is looking forward in an optimistic, proactive manner. People around her treat her as they did before the stroke. In not changing their behavior, Georgia's friends and relatives aren't showing her disrespect, nor are they indifferent to her plight. Rather, they indicate that they respect what she has already accomplished and what she hopes to accomplish. In showing this respect for her capacity and willpower, they encourage her to do things on her own—even though it must be difficult to watch her struggle with her disabled body.

Family members and friends often face nearly as great a challenge as the stroke survivor in terms of shifting realities. Partners who have looked forward to foreign travel or shared hobbies when they and their spouse retire must now look forward to spending the rest of their lives as caregivers. This experience can be devastating. Children who have begun their own independent lives must now devote at least some of their free time to taking care of their invalid parents. Parents of younger survivors, such as Rod, must confront the prospect of an active parental role for many more years than they had anticipated. People who are used to playing bridge with their good friend must now either abandon their bridge games or find a new bridge partner, given the inability of this friend to speak or hold cards.

What is the impact of poststroke recovery on relationships with the family members and friends of those we interviewed? And how can professional caregivers help all the parties involved adjust to the new realities?

Family Members

Mary indicated during her interview that she is angry not only because she can't write as easily or clearly as she used to but also because people around her every day treat her differently now. She is particularly galled that she can't do the dishes (a chore that she felt trusted to do before her stroke). Mary said that her family worries a lot and tends to treat her as if she's become fragile and requires constant attention.

Sheila also perceives that people treat her differently. Her estranged husband felt she should be committed to a nursing home because he thought she was mentally disabled. The reactions of her children were varied. Her sons did everything for her during the recovery process, but she would not allow them to treat her like a child. Her oldest son seemed committed to taking her home to live with his brother and himself, but Sheila wanted to return to her own home. Her two daughters were in shock after the stroke and found it difficult to cope with the ensuing family crisis. They initially avoided being around Sheila but later tried, like her sons, to treat her as a child. One of Sheila's sons describes the stroke as having a profound impact on each member of the family. Today, Sheila's children harbor resentment, and conflict exists regarding the way each of them initially coped with the crisis and the way they continue to react to their mother. Sheila thinks her children need support even more than she does. She is optimistic about herself and strives to find ways to feel productive. She only wishes that her children could resolve their own sibling problems.

Susan has also had to grapple with the changing perceptions of others. Her husband became very frustrated that she wasn't the same person; he didn't want to confront the fact that she now was more fragile than she had been before her stroke. He became angry and frustrated because she could no longer hold a job or keep up with the housework. Susan finally divorced her demanding husband after she almost lost her life during one of his physical assaults on her. This man had to change if he was to continue in a relationship with his wife. The demands that he made were never equitable or realistic. However, they became even more outlandish after Susan had her stroke. Something had to give— either Susan's continuing recovery or their long-term marriage. Fortunately, Susan no longer agreed to be a victim.

But she also encountered difficulties with other family members. Her father initially reacted to her poststroke physical condition by concluding that "she does not remember anything," when in fact her major problem was one of short-term memory and communication. Her father's attitude was very frustrating, for Susan had a clear memory of things that had happened a long time ago. She doesn't like being treated like a child by her family and finds that this patronizing treatment is often based on the untested assumption that she can't do something or has become "stupid."

As is the case with the friends and relatives of many stroke survivors, Susan's family made the incorrect assumption that her loss of cognitive skills (such as short-term memory) indicates the loss of many other related skills. It is so easy for those of us who have not had strokes to allow our presuppositions and fears to govern our own actions and our relationships with the stroke survivor. One of the people doing the interviews, for instance, reflected on her own preconceptions in beginning the first interview with a stroke survivor: "My immediate reaction to Jane on our meeting was that of relief. Relief because she presented herself as quite verbal, open, and she engaged well with me. She appeared high-functioning, involved in many activities including golf, dancing, and entertaining in her home. Her home was filled with activity—grandchildren playing, her son visiting, the telephone ringing— and she had a full schedule for the weekend. I had anticipated a somewhat frail, isolated, depressed person with cognitive/speech limitations. Unfortunately, that was my own preconceived notion of stroke survivors."

The physical damage done by a stroke is often quite localized, and the extent of dysfunction following a stroke varies dramatically from one survivor to the next. The psychological damage done by misguided preconceptions and untested assumptions about the lost capacities and limited opportunities of survivors, on the other hand, can lead to general and lasting damage in impeding the recovery of self-esteem and self-empowerment. Those of us who have not had strokes must check our own preconceptions at the door when meeting stroke survivors or, like the insightful interviewer, must be willing to let our preconceived notions change as we interact with a specific person who is coping with a stroke in a unique and often admirable manner.

Susan shares with Rod, Sheila, and many other stroke survivors the difficult experience of being stared at in public. She has adjusted to the strange looks from people in her community and is fully aware that she now speaks more slowly than the average person and that she sometimes loses track of what she is talking about. Strangers are going to arrive at the conclusion that she is slow or even in some sense retarded. Her family, however, should know better. Like many stroke survivors, Susan wishes they would treat her as a mature, competent adult.

Since her stroke, Carla feels greater confidence in asking for and doing what she wants instead of what others want her to do. She has arrived at this state largely because of inadequacies in the assistance she has received from others around her—in particular, her husband. Carla suggested that since her stroke, people sometimes treat her as if she doesn't have a brain. Her husband is especially inclined to tell her what to do—even more than before the stroke. "People tell you what to do, what to wear, but no one can tell me what to think." In many ways, Carla has become more assertive since the stroke, while at the same time, her husband and others have become increasingly controlling. She thinks that this new assertiveness has hurt her marriage. Her husband was an accountant who retired in 1989. So, just as he moved into his own transition from work to retirement, he also had to face the transition of taking care of his disabled wife.

Carla claimed that her husband has made other plans for their life, but he has not talked with her about these plans. When she tries to broach the subject, he refuses to talk. Her husband has to do most of the cooking and cleaning. Unlike Susan's husband, he has accepted this new reality. However, communication between Carla and her husband has deteriorated since her stroke, in part because of these additional responsibilities. He now always seems to be busy and has little time to spend with her.

Carla believes that her husband has some negative feelings about her and the stroke; however, he won't talk about them. She thinks it would be easier if he did communicate—though like many males, he finds communication about personal feelings difficult. He does go with her to a stroke club, but she noted that neither has the freedom to express feelings openly since the other is always there. Her husband has no other support group. She wishes he had a place to talk without her. Carla thinks that he wants both to take care of her and to control her and that he feels tied down by her. She firmly believes that his feelings are justified, since he spends most of his time taking care of her. According to her, there are too many unsaid things between them. She assumes that he blames her, and wishes that he would express his anger.

Carla is glad that her husband is active, even though retired. He meets with a client several times each week, and Carla feels this is a good thing. He gets away from her, and she gets some free time without him hovering around. Since the stroke, her husband has refused to have sex with her and she misses this. He doesn't talk to her about this either. Like many women, Carla tries to communicate when she feels disconnected. Like many men, her husband pulls away from this request for intimacy and engagement, finding this to be a threat to his need for autonomy. Unfortunately, this all-too-common pattern of male-female communication leaves the female stroke survivor with little support from her spouse precisely when she most needs reassurance, empathy, and understanding.

Her interviewer observed that the distance between Carla and her husband is not a figment of Carla's imagination. The interviewer felt uncomfortable with the husband. While he was in the house during the interview, she could clearly not speak openly about her feelings of being "a nobody." As soon as he left, however, she spoke freely. So even though she reported feeling more assertive, there was evidence that she still isn't very assertive toward her husband. Is she really more independent, or just less comfortable in being dependent on him? How would her husband have responded had he been asked about his perception of Carla's behavior since the stroke? Has her stroke changed the balance of power (or at least the pattern of assertiveness) in the household? Can she now feel more in control? In the long run, is it likely that both partners will be pleased with the shift in the relationship? These remain unanswered questions in Carla's marriage and in the marriages of other survivors who have become more (or less) assertive as a result of their stroke.

Carla's children do not live close by, further exacerbating the problem. She feels that they are somewhat closer to her since the stroke, but she doesn't see them very often, and they have not really talked about the stroke much at all. She believes that stroke survivors generally want to talk about their condition but that people who are close to them often don't. She may be quite accurate with regard to many female stroke survivors, though other stroke survivors (both female and male) often are seeking more autonomy and don't particularly want to spend much time talking about their problems. Those who do want to talk are often much better off than those who remain isolated.

Given that many of those who don't want to talk are males, the real challenge for those working with stroke survivors may often be to get the male survivors to somehow open up communication with significant people in their lives (wife, children, friends), who are usually eager to be helpful. Carla was pleased to be able to participate in the interview, for it was "good to get some of these things out." For Carla and many other women (and some men) we interviewed, "there is no one else to tell them to." But in some cases, talking (especially excessive talking) can create problems rather than provide healing. Some stroke survivors try to evoke pity in everyone they meet and appear to almost delight in telling stories of suffering and loss. These survivors often seem to turn the stroke itself as well as stories of the stroke into weapons that they are using to strike out against people around them who have not had strokes.

Most stroke survivors, however, do not wallow in self-pity. They often do not talk enough about their experiences and feel isolated. As in the case with many women we interviewed (such as Susan and Carla),

Thelma found her husband of "no help" in her adaptation to the post-stroke conditions in her life. He certainly was not someone she could talk to. When she was discharged from the hospital, her husband took her home and helped her with "physical things." However, like Carla's husband, he couldn't talk about the stroke with her and seemed to feel uncomfortable if she tried to bring it up.

Thelma's husband refused to read any of the material about the stroke that the hospital provided, and when he was invited to a "family support group," he refused to attend. Thelma's husband now spends most of his free time playing golf and remains reluctant to talk about her stroke. She can't even turn to her children for support. She denies that she has been angry about her husband's reactions to her stroke, saying that "Clifton was never one to empathize" and that she was not surprised at his reaction. With regard to her children, Thelma rationalized that "my children were grown [when I had my stroke] and already had their own lives."

Thelma was surprised at the reactions of most of her friends—an experience that has left her bitter. She reported that many of them stopped calling or visiting and that she has completely lost touch with most of them. Her impression is that "most people are scared of you when you've had a stroke" and that "you really find out who your friends are when something like this happens." She thought she had many friends but now believes that she has only "two or three real friends." Thelma gets her greatest satisfaction from giving practical advice to other stroke survivors at the stroke club and her local "Y."

Apparently the people who have been closest to Thelma let her down at a crucial point in her life. They were unwilling to face the reality of the stroke, to make changes in their own lives, or to make their relationship with Thelma a high priority. As a result, she is left with little support from others and must find solace not by receiving assistance, but rather by helping others who have recently had strokes. While the act of offering help to others is better than nothing, one can't resist feeling angry and sad for Thelma regarding the failure of both her friends and family. Her friends certainly have a right to separate from her, though one wonders what true friendship really is if people are going to leave us during hard times. Her husband and children, however, who Thelma expects to be of minimal assistance, do have an obligation to be supportive of her during this difficult transition. The value of any family is most clearly exemplified at a time like this in the life of one of its members.

Other stroke survivors—unlike Thelma—found that their stroke brought out the best in their mate. Marriages have been solidified. New levels of intimacy and mutuality have been attained. Alice said that her husband "is like an angel" and has been very supportive of her, as have her sons and friends. She retired from the military seven years ago but still keeps in touch with her friends, who have remained with her despite her retirement and stroke. Todd similarly reported that he received strong support from family members, particularly his wife, on whom he seems to depend because of his loss of memory after the stroke. Throughout his interview, he spoke positively of the support he has received from family and friends, as well as emphasizing the importance of his support group and the role this support has played in his progress toward recovery. He greatly appreciates being able to maintain an ongoing positive relationship with his wife.

Todd seemed to be quite aware of how his relationship with his wife, close friends, and students have changed. It was important to him to be treated with sensitivity by others, but not to the point of being looked at as being different or excluded from an activity simply because he was perceived as too fragile to handle it. He seems to be asking for just about the same thing as most of the other men and women we interviewed—what we have called the delicate balance between challenge and support. He recalls being made aware of this balancing act occasionally when friends forget and catch themselves asking him to do something that he is no longer capable of (too much challenge and not enough support) or when they overcompensate (not enough challenge and too much support).

Todd seems to have little difficulty making people aware of his situation. When asked how he felt about having to explain to others why he might not be able to perform certain tasks well within the reach of other people at his age and station in life, he said, "I know where

I am with this." He went on to explain that if he were to tell someone that he couldn't read, he would prefer to tell them why—that it was due to his stroke. Todd strongly believes that he would much rather tell someone about his disability than have them assume that he never learned to read. Immediately after his stroke, he was only capable of reading at a second-grade level.

Todd was diligent in his rehabilitation efforts and eventually recovered these cherished cognitive skills. He returned to work after five months and teaches at a neighborhood college. He believes that giving people information about his stroke and disability can be helpful in allowing them to better understand his situation. While some stroke survivors try to hide the existence and cause of their disability for fear that other people will avoid them, patronize them, or assume that they are totally disabled, Todd takes a logical and adaptive stance in meeting new people—he is quick to tell them about himself.

Friends

In our interviews, we found that many stroke survivors relied primarily on the support offered by their friends, since their spouse, children, or other family members either were not present or, like Thelma's and Susan's family, were not helpful. In some cases, friends have been of greatest value when they continue to relate to the stroke survivor as if nothing has happened. Betsy feels that the important friends in her life have treated her the same as they did prior to her stroke. She was very active before the stroke and felt at first that she would not be able to participate in the same groups and organizations. Her friends did not change their expectations, however, and called her anyway.

Betsy has continued to see them and is active in two organizations and a sorority. The executive board of one of the organizations meets in her home, and she prepares food for the meeting in addition to assuming regular committee duties. She is also able to attend the annual debutante ball given by her sorority and regularly attends church. She and her friends all believe that she is going to live a long life, and they encourage her to do what she can with the time she has. Betsy enjoys getting out of her house and visiting with friends and family. She also has a positive relationship with her occupational and physical therapists and knows that they have been important in her recovery. Unlike some of the people we interviewed, she seems to have an abundance of sensitive, thoughtful, and caring friends and professional assistants in her life. With such support, she is undoubtedly justified in expecting a long, event-filled life.

Many stroke survivors and their friends are less fortunate. As we've seen, the stroke experience often puts close relationships to the test, and not all friends are willing or able to be more patient, more supportive, more sensitive, or more accepting of mood swings and limitations in the range of activities that they can share with the survivor. The very essence of a friendship is often challenged at the point that a stroke survivor asks for help from a long-term friend. Is this really a friendship that will survive the stroke or, hopefully, actually grow richer as a result of the support that the friend provides?

The latter is certainly the case for Greta. She attributes much of her successful recovery to her supportive friends (as well as the helpful professionals who have encouraged her). Greta has met new people who have helped her, as have her long-term friends. By participating in a stroke support group, she has been able to both give and receive assistance. She has always loved being with people, and she continues to regularly see longtime friends, participate in social activities that suit her new life-style, and travel with friends when she can. After her interview, Greta was about to fly to Boston to see another friend. This was going to be the first time she has flown alone since her stroke, though friends were going to take her to the airport and others will pick her up. A wonderful balance between support and challenge was offered by her friends. We should all be so fortunate!

Sheila's experience has been more ambivalent. She said that some of her friends treat her the same as before her stroke. She is still included, for example, in social events, such as dinner shows. This has helped her gain a sense of normalcy. Other friends, however, felt uncomfortable around her and broke off their relationship with her. As in the case of Rod McLean, the reactions of strangers have often been difficult to take. The often-rude responses of adults in public tend to irritate Sheila—especially when they tell their children not to stare. Sheila thinks it's healthy for children to want to ask questions so that they can learn that disabled people are not to be feared.

John feels that he must rely pretty much on himself in recovering from his stroke. Furthermore, recovery has been a long and difficult process—in part because of what he perceives as the failure of friends to be there for him. John remains outraged that it took a year before he received any home nursing support or physical therapy. In addition, he feels "let down" by his friends and his church. He believes that the only reason many of his friends and fellow church members came to his aid was out of a sense of duty, not love. As a result, John no longer attends church and does his worshipping at home alone. He claims that the number of people he can call friends has dropped dramatically.

John continues to have contact with one or two people he cares for but spends most of his time alone. He states that this is not a problem for him, since he is content using "fantasy" to occupy his mind and pass the time. He probably helped to set the stage for his alienation from people who used to be important to him. He may have expected too much from his friends and made it difficult for them to show their love and affection. Some stroke survivors, like John, interpret the expression of concern and support by friends as nothing more than obligation or even a condescending "going through the motions." These survivors often can't avail themselves of the assistance offered and soon become isolated and bitter.

Jim and Tom are among those who seem to be alienated from people who probably want to help them. However, they are not so much worried about condescension as they are about the burden they place on those who live with and around them. Jim mentioned several times during his interview that no one believes he has had a stroke because nothing "looks different." He is not alone among stroke survivors in struggling with the "invisibility" of his disability. While strangers might not know of the stroke, the experience of having a stroke and recovering from it is burned forever on any survivor's memory. The survivor will never be the same, even if the source of the radical change is unknown to most people. Jim's relatives are well aware of major differences in his ability to perform many tasks. They know the source of the changes in his life. While Jim does not tell anyone new to his life that he has had a stroke, the people who do know him—especially members of his family—bother him because he is sensitive to the problems he causes and wants to retain his independence.

Tom's disabilities are more noticeable than Jim's. Tom said that people in his community no longer stop and chat, and he assumes that they think he is a bit odd. This is difficult for him, because he had always been active and respected in his community. Closer to home, however, the problems for Tom appear to be even more serious and resemble those faced by Jim. In a whisper (so that his son couldn't hear), Tom indicated to his interviewer: "I guess I'm stuck here with her [pointing to the house where his wife was] and with him [nodding toward his son]." He feels his own constrictions in not easily being able to leave his home, but even more keenly feels what the constraints must be like for his wife and son. When discussing how he manages this difficult situation, he stated, "I just take it a day at a time. That's all I can do." Like many stroke survivors we interviewed, Tom sees many problems in his near future and tries to consider and plan for this future in small units ("one day at a time") so that the prospects of being confined for many years with his wife and son don't overwhelm him.

We have seen in all of these case studies of stroke survivors that the support of other people is critical. This is not a good time in one's life to be going it alone. Other people are needed for physical assistance and running errands and—most important—for encouraging and appreciating one's rehabilitation efforts. In earlier time periods, most people had nearby extended families or at least longtime neighbors and friends on whom they could rely for this support. Today, unfortunately, many stroke survivors do not have these more "natural" support networks. Together with those friends and family members who are available, stroke survivors must purposefully create their own support network. Stroke clubs often are an invaluable component of this network. Other community, church, and recreational agencies can also be of great benefit, even if they are not specifically geared to stroke survivors. The

services provided should be thoughtfully conceived and ultimately controlled by the survivors so that both challenge and support are offered
at appropriate times and places.

Professional Caregivers

Professional caregivers are often just as guilty of insensitivity as friends
and family regarding the self-esteem of stroke survivors. Much as Rod
describes in confronting an apparently well-intentioned counselor, the
professional caregiver who assumes a condescending or pessimistic and
limiting attitude with reference to stroke survivors often is doing more
harm than good in treating them. We find that survivors and caregivers
often come in for counseling after being disappointed with the treatment they received at other facilities. One stroke survivor (whom we
will call Ted) and his wife, Bea, for instance, were discouraged with
the speech therapist at one facility, where he was told that he would
never be able to speak intelligibly. Ted contacted another facility and
was assigned to a wonderful and competent speech therapist, who worked
with him for many months. He has improved with her guidance and
determination. Ted came to a stroke support group after several months
of therapy. Like Rod, Ted was embarrassed by his aphasia; however,
he was determined to say his name and did so after several minutes.
He also said "good morning." He deeply moved the group with his
courage and perseverance. The entire group clapped for him that day
in acknowledgment of his achievement. Caregivers—both professional
and personal—must always be vigilant regarding assumptions and expectations. Stroke survivors can perform miracles, if given a chance.

In other instances, the problem is not the insensitivity of health
care providers, but simply the absence of any follow-up services for stroke
survivors. They are constantly confronted out in the world by the fear,
disgust, and discouragement of other people who know little about
strokes or about recovery from strokes. We must often provide follow-
up services as a way of giving stroke survivors (and their families) a boost.
Pete, for instance, had initially been at a hospital that had no outpatient program. After leaving the hospital, he received some home phys-

ical therapy for a few months, but nothing after that. His wife called the rehabilitation center, looking for a support group and more medical assistance. He was readily and happily accepted into the support group. During the first week, Pete and his social worker discussed his regression in walking (he came to the group in a wheelchair), and the social worker suggested a reevaluation. He was reevaluated and entered physical therapy for about six weeks. He soon began coming to group by walking with a one-pronged cane and entered the pool therapy class. Hope has been restored to Pete and his family for continued progress.

Care is expressed in a variety of ways with regard to work with stroke survivors. We need to ensure that they don't become isolated and that appropriate services are made available to them. We should also be sure that they have received adequate information and know that various forms of support are available, if they need them. Truly helpful care, however, is not always expressed by lending a hand; it is often more thoughtfully expressed through not lending a hand—through letting stroke survivors do it on their own with the encouragement, support, and understanding of caregivers. Care is also expressed by examining personal biases and assumptions when first meeting or working with stroke survivors. All too frequently, a caregiver's expectations are self-fulfilling—just as a survivor's expectations are self-fulfilling. Many expect survivors to be feeble of mind or body and, by relating to them in a patronizing, overbearing way, we foster their dependency on us or even force them to lose their own will to overcome their disability. When we assume that stroke survivors can't do something or shouldn't try to accomplish something, we also exhibit our lack of respect for them and, as a result, possibly contribute to their own loss of self-esteem—which is the most devastating and long-lasting of all disabilities!

PART THREE

Reentering the World

9

Returning Home

When we got to the family's house, everyone piled out as I (Rod McLean) tried to get out, too. As I was being helped out of the car, Linda presented me with a carved wooden cane. She was remarkably caring and proud of me. I accepted and appreciated the "crutch." I gazed at the front door of the house. From the car to the door never looked so far before. I glanced at my friends and family: "By myself!" They all respected my determination to do it alone. It took a while— the seconds were hours! The rough cement pathway was slightly inclined and had a couple of cracks; it also had two steep stairs. Parallel balance bars had not yet been installed along the path. At the top, I leaned the cane against the house and reached to open the door, then stopped and remembered that I was going to have to use my right hand as much as possible. I still had to mechanically control the damaged muscles—and would always have to.

We all moseyed into the family room and enjoyed each other's company for a while. Linda then whispered to me, "Let's go! I want to show you something you might like!" and winked at me. We got into her car and she started talking about a million things as we pulled into traffic. I wondered where we were going and felt her hand softly squeezing my thigh. She turned into a side street, stopped the car, and pulled the emergency brake. She immediately kissed and embraced me strongly, reminding me how long it had been. "We're going to my place; it will be the best!" My innocent and slow mind was wondering, "What might 'it' be?" But within a second, my other brain understood and came to attention for service! I was excited! After the immediate thrill, my psyche was taken over with a dark cloud of questions and apprehensiveness about my ability to "perform." "My God, I've wanted this opportunity since I came out of my coma . . . do my 'tools' work? . . . can I satisfy her? . . . am I agile enough? . . . can I endure? . . . am I only half a person? . . . or am I still okay?" As we parked, entered the house, and went into the bedroom, my heart and brain were throbbing. I was continuing to pop questions about my manhood and sexual identity—the backbone to my personality and my key to normality!

My anxiety was peaking until her soft lips touched mine. We eased into ecstasy for the rest of the afternoon and into the night. I lay with her and my ego came back, even though I was disabled. As I rested with her in my arms, I gained another feather for my cap; I thought that now I could take the world on as a person.

The next morning I got ready for the day, but after a moment I realized that I hadn't planned anything. I stared angrily at my new dress shoes, because the right shoe had been "orthopedicized" with a huge, clanky, metal half-calf ankle brace. I sputtered, complained, and threatened to toss out this gross symbol of being "handicapped." I hated it all! I especially hated the fact that with every right-footed step I took, the brace made a loud iron clunk! With each of the million steps I was to take, this sound would remind me of my unwanted new identity.

"Damn!" Well, anyhow . . . I'm so happy to leave the hospital and return to freedom. I think I'd like to step out into the neighborhood and try my first posthospital exercise. I'm going to attempt to walk around the block. I set a plan, visualized the action, looked at my feet, and commanded them to get going! I had a hard time keeping everything coordinated and also seeing where I was going; most of the time I had to continue watching and commanding my legs and feet, but every so often I raised my eyes to gauge the checkpoints. I looked to see how far it was to the end of the block. It was forever, and there were no parallel bars! How far to each house and how far to each forty-inch form line on the sidewalk? Sometimes it felt like I was in a groove; at other moments, I felt awkward and almost fell. Eventually, I made it all the way to the end of the block.

It was demanding and took so long, but a nice distraction was that some of the neighbors came out of their houses to say "hi!", "good having you back," or just acknowledging that I was still living. "Thanks!" Even though I had to concentrate on my body's movement, I was feeling great! I was breathing it in! I felt that I was on a roll! "Yeah, I think . . . actually, I know I can go all the way around the block!" I set my plan and started around the corner, up a very mild hill. As I started down the other side, I discovered wonderful symbols of living in America. I was totally exhilarated!

I spotted three little kids across the street playing marbles. One of the kids, probably seven years old or so, was squatting and was just about to shoot his cat-eye at one of the other marbles. I could tell when he was cocking and shooting to win by seeing him with his tongue in his cheek! "What a simple and insignificant scenario, but what a rich and momentous thing for me to experience! This tells me how much of a miracle it is that I'm alive!" All of a sudden, as I was enjoying the moment, one of the kids looked over in my direction, pointed, and yelled, "Yikes! He's weird!" They forgot the marbles and ran away.

I looked behind me expecting to see a gross, scary monster, but I realized there was no one around me at all. Slowly and painfully, I became aware that the kids were frightened of *me*! I became light-headed, my face felt flushed, and my whole body shook. I caught my balance. "They're teasing me! They're making fun of me!" I was devastated. Watching the children was a great source of joy, but now my soul was shriveling from anguish. I was humiliated by the kids teasing me. Their ignorance had shattered my reality. Even though I was still Rod, I appeared different. I was trying to expel the anger and pain. "Why do I have to go through this? Why me? God, this hurts! Why didn't this happen to someone who deserved it?" As I was displacing my pain, I wished I could have the kids come back, sit down, and listen to my story of being an okay person. I wanted them to know that my "package" had tumbled and now has some dents—that's how simple it was.

However, there were two major problems: the kids were gone, and I could barely speak at that time! I just sputtered with frustration for a while, then a thought started crystallizing: "You know, in actuality, I was supposed to die, but I lived anyhow . . . some people have said that it was a miracle. But miracles have to have profound purposes . . . what's my mission? . . . if I can get my previous capacities—or even just some of them—back, like the ability to speak and to physically get around, I could do so much. And I want people to understand that I'm still a person! I can advocate for myself; I can empower myself! . . . and maybe if I get it together, I can help other people face the same experiences. People might seem odd by being limited, but they are still human beings with the same emotions and beliefs as everyone else. If that's what the miracle is all about, I'm not going to lose sight of that idea. I want to teach children about life; I want to use my experiences as a window for people to see and understand those who are different."

I continued thinking in that vein and realized that I needed to get around the corner. I felt I had to get home. I still felt light-headed; I had to regain my focus, organize my thoughts, produce a plan, and put it into action. As I looked around to get my bearings, everything looked so far away. But I knew it was manageable if I would just shelve those abstract thoughts while focusing on more mundane mechanical tasks like trying to walk the whole way home. When I finally got home and settled down, I did return to what I'd been thinking about earlier. I was convinced that all this did have a purpose.

Even after I'd been out of the hospital for a couple of months, everything moved slowly and took me so long to get done. I had to retrain myself to do every minuscule thing I took for granted; everything had to be rebuilt from scratch. Sometimes I thought I was stuck in low gear and couldn't double-clutch into the next gear. Every day I performed a set of specific stretches and flexes that the physical therapist had worked out for me. Every day I practiced and increased my walking distance and endurance. Outpatient physical therapy, speech therapy, occupational therapy, swimming, and exercise at the YMCA were set up for me. I even decided to take some college classes.

Gradually, I began to be reoriented and settled into a bit of normality. I figured out schedules so that I could attend all my therapeutic sessions by bus. Most of the therapies were on Tuesday and Thursday, which were long days. Much of the time, a member of my family would give me a ride to the first session, then I would walk a couple of blocks to the next session and then on to the next, until the last one. I was very close to a bus stop. During the first couple of weeks, I did take the bus home. It went about seven miles and let me out about half a block from the house. "Wasn't that convenient?" From the first step up into the bus I watched my feet moving correctly, but felt something very uncomfortable. As I grasped the standing pole for stability, I raised my eyes and noticed people looking at me. They quickly glanced away to avoid their own uncomfortable reactions. It felt just the same as the little kids who teased me and offered me my first negative experience outside of the hospital.

"God, I hate that pain!" I felt like jumping in the faces of these passengers on the bus. I wanted to square up, nose to nose, and scream at them, "I may be different, but I'm still alive and I'm okay." When I feel that specific way, my whole physical body cringes. The muscles tighten up and become even more uncomfortable and less coordinated. Again, "I hate this vulnerable feeling." For a couple of weeks, I did continue busing, even though I didn't like it. When I was riding, I tried to watch and focus on whatever I was passing by, but internally I was uncomfortable, angry, and frustrated and wanting to get off the bus and run away from my disability role. One day, I completed the last session, walked out of the building, and glanced across the street—only to see the bus departing. In the following thirty minutes, I tried to figure out a solution. "How about running after the bus and racing up to it? Ha! . . . Wait for the next bus? Nah, it takes too long and I don't accept relying on something that reminds me of my limits. Phone home? Nah, I want to be more independent." Then I tried hitchhiking for a while with no success. "So, I think I'll just walk for a while and see how it goes."

I looked at each foot stepping forward. When I got some rhythm going, I was able to think about more than just the physical movement. I planned for the future. I analyzed what I had experienced, about the way it used to be. I reviewed how it could be. I practiced mental games, did calisthenics with my memory, repeated many speech drills, and rehearsed my college assignments. Every so often, I would look up and register where I was. I would take a break from concentration and observe what was going on around me at the time, until I'd stumble. Immediately, the thought of giving up flashed in front of me, but I had to react to each falter by strengthening my determination! Then I had to get back on track. A couple of hours later, I dragged into the house carrying a big smile of accomplishment in climbing another impossible plateau!

My rehabilitation experiences were intense; when they were completed, I was a happy camper. At the beginning of the year-long speech therapy process, I sat face to face with the therapist while he showed me hundreds of pen-and-ink drawings of common objects. These included a knife, table, car, chair, newspaper, door, checkbook, television set, dinner plate, lamp, bed, and so forth; I had to name each of them. It was so frustrating. I instantly recognized each object, but as soon as I tried to say its name, I would lose the concept! "How did that happen?" You know it's right there; then you reach for it, and it's gone! Everyone, at one time or another, has forgotten a specific word: "It's right on the tip of my tongue!" Imagine what it would be like if not just one word or phrase were inaccessible, but the entire 30,000 to 50,000 words in your vocabulary. Sometimes I couldn't access a single one of them, no matter how hard I tried. "Frustration" is the nicest word for the experience. It's as if all of one's linguistic knowledge is stored in a four-drawer filing cabinet. Imagine that some elves sneak into the office, knock the filing cabinet over, and then strew the documents all over the floor. My language capacity had absolutely no structure or organization; every time I wanted to utter a word, I had to get on my knees and look through all the millions of document sheets in the mess. I knew what word I wanted to find and to say, but by the time I found it, either I'd forgotten what the subject was or the other person had already walked away. Another analogy is between your brain and a computer. The ultra-powered PC is all programmed, structured, and networked so its synapses are just popping, when there is a major overload. One of the results is that the computer chip for communication is scorched. There's a glitch. Every time I use that program, it shorts out. Thus, I must completely rewire the program with no materials or tools!

By practicing and repeating with those baby-level cards for a month, I responded to all 300 cards perfectly! It seemed to take forever to figure out some of the drawings, but I was more stubborn than the aphasia. Sometimes it took me a lot of time; the speech therapist could have left, done grocery shopping, gotten a haircut, and caught up on some calls and would have still had a minute to help me out. But I wouldn't give up. I practiced not only at the clinic, but all the time. At times, everything I would see, I would say aloud, and after many months, I would say it silently just to practice. After the cards were accomplished, we would start on other language tasks; we immediately attacked the next, larger, and more ferocious monsters to slay. When we completed a task, we'd start working on the next plan; with the cards, we were just connecting sounds to the symbols, then putting the small words together to produce a statement or sentence, then practicing abstract concepts, larger sentences, sentence structure, and redeveloping my personal thesaurus. We totally reprogrammed my expressive and receptive communication system. Throughout the year, we did all sorts of different projects that demanded most of my language capacity. Toward the ninth month of the speech therapy sessions, the therapist and I developed a light personal friendship. It seemed that he cared about my progress and wanted me to do as well as possible. In a trusting way, I felt that the sessions became even richer and more powerful. We were more in tune with each other and understood how the other worked. He learned the best ways for me to put it all back together, and I learned more about him so that I could trust him to let him do an even better job of teaching me.

This went on intensively for twelve months. At the fiftieth week of sessions, he explained that we only had fifty-two weeks of therapy according to the terms of the insurance policy. "And you have done more than anyone could even imagine; you have gone past anything we could have anticipated." At the same time, I knew that I was barely above the survival level. I only had developed access to maybe 500 words in my vocabulary. The therapist tried to explain that I had accomplished everything the clinic could offer. We worked even harder to finish the last session on a crescendo of emotion. During the last five minutes of our final meeting, the therapist expressed how great it had been. It was not only that he had helped me a lot, but he also said he had learned so much from me as a stroke survivor. By knowing me, he now knows how to help all the survivors that he expects to work with in his professional life. He also indicated that we had developed a friendship. "Rod, from right now, what do you want to do in your life? What schooling? What type of work? . . . "

I reviewed my interests. I started to feel overwhelmed and warm as I approached the topic of teaching children with disabilities. It felt right. The spark of excitement is starting to flame! In my aphasically slow and drawling manner, I sheepishly stuttered, "I . . . I . . . uh . . . I think . . . well . . . you know . . . I really feel . . . I want to *teach!* To teach children. To help them to understand." I paused. I glanced at the therapist. He had been leaning forward to understand what I was trying to portray. His initial facial language was saying that he was supportive and caring. Within a half second, when his brain grasped specifically what I was expressing, he showed shock and fear. He gulped, tried to control being flustered. He gathered himself, looked at me, paused, and started, "Rod, . . . you had a severe stroke! The aneurysm massively damaged the communication area!" His voice became stronger and louder. "The most important requirement in teaching is being strong in communication. You have to be very fluent: speaking, reading, writing, explaining! . . . Rod, *you cannot teach!*"

I felt devastated! I felt violated! My new excitement was shattered! I was betrayed! My anger seeped to the surface and shifted into pure rage! My "feelings barriers" shot up. I hid my emotions, tightened my jaw, curled my lips inwardly, and with an invincible poker face, stood up, quickly shook his hand, sputtered "thanks" under my breath, and attempted to stumble proudly out of the office. When I opened the clinic's heavy glass door to the outside, I quickly and deeply sucked in the crisp October air. I stood for a moment composing myself. As I began walking to my next session—in occupational therapy—I had to concentrate on my leg movements. However, I was constantly distracted by my throbbing and exploding emotions!

The fact that my therapist told me that I couldn't do something I wanted to do irritated me for years. For a while, it was a heavy burden to carry around all the time. I went back to college two months after I got out of the hospital. My goal and purpose at college, at that time, was still very basic. Shortly after the speech therapy program's termination, I crystallized my plan to teach people with disabilities. I then used the therapist's expressed "ceiling" as my spur to do the impossible. I was going to be a severely aphasic stroke survivor who became a teacher! In fact, I attended college for many years, and later had the opportunity to confront my speech therapist. I was sitting on a bench at a mall in front of a large department store waiting for my fiancée to get off work. While I was waiting, I was just watching people. From a distance, I recognized my old speech therapist. As he approached, he recognized me, too. "Rod! . . . Rod McLean! . . . How are you doing? You look good . . . " "It's good to see you, too . . . ," I acknowledged. "Well, what are you doing nowadays? Are you working at a sheltered workshop? . . . Are you going to school?" I nodded. "Are you still a freshman?" "No." "A sophomore?" "No." "Are you still attending junior college?" "No!" "Are you a junior now?" He expressed greater anxiety. "No." "Rod, would you please tell me what you are doing?" "Yes! A few years ago, I got my B.A. degree (the same level you achieved, right?). My major was psychology. Currently, I am attending the University of Washington . . . working toward a master's degree in special education. This program is one of the top five in the United States—one of the most competitive, too. Most of my work is *teaching!*" (Phil paused and looked at the tips of his shoes.) I let it sit for what must have seemed forever, but most likely was about half a minute. I saw his temples flexing and moistening.

When he looked up at me again, I slowly began, "I'm not a vindictive person . . . but I've been waiting and working toward this moment for years! Right now, I'm relishing it. I know back then you tried to help me with reality. And your intentions were good, and your reference point was from all the information that you had accumulated from the college texts. But do you know . . . do you realize what you hadn't taken into account? That you had forgotten the most important ingredient? You forgot about the individual you were serving. Yes, the books explained the situation to the readers in general, but it's generic . . . it's approximate . . . it's most likely, but it isn't *me!* And every new "patient" is not and never will be generic. They all are unique and special and always deserve every possible option. They should never be unnecessarily limited!" We kept up the eye contact. I turned my volume down. "I do thank you for everything." Then we shook hands. I felt completed and noticed Linda looking for me. She and I saluted the experience. I floated on a cloud to embrace her, and then explained my new satisfaction.

When I was out of the hospital, I was trying to reorient myself and reevaluate, readapt, readjust, and restructure virtually everything about myself. Some things were simple, but many were difficult and many more appeared impossible. One of the difficulties I didn't imagine ever happening was that my relationship with Linda eventually went sour. When we were starting the relationship, we were happy and saw everything through rose-colored glasses. We wanted to hold hands and skip into the sunset. Not quite! A bit before my stroke, reality had started seeping into our fantasy world. When the stroke happened, the truth rushed in! I think for quite a while, we tried to outrun our problems: we rationalized, we tried to get to the basics, and we attempted to put a false veneer on what was really going on. Our pretty world was cracking and the loose ends were unraveling. When the stroke happened, Linda was there. While I was in the hospital, she was there with support, without question. But when I was released and we began making our way back into the real world, that was where our life was tested—and got testy. Over time, the fibers that made up the weave of our relationship got more and more frayed, and eventually, they snapped. God, this sounds like an ordinary relationship! You know, it just went its course—we went in other directions, our viewpoints changed, and the affection and caring were lost. At times we tried to recapture the feelings we thought we'd had. But there were other times I hardly knew her as the person she used to be with me.

To be honest, when I think of all I went through, I realize I was especially afraid of losing her because she was my connection to being "normal." Deep inside, I thought poorly of myself and was terrified of losing someone's love, even if it wasn't really unconditional. I thought if a person rejected me, nobody would love me because I felt much less than a whole person. It was scary to feel so insecure. Even though we never spoke about it, I believe she had major difficulties shifting her feelings to the new person I was—someone she didn't know or even want to try giving a chance to. It was possible she couldn't completely accept a "damaged" person. She may have realized she couldn't go the full distance. It could have been that she was afraid of being embarrassed by me or my disability. Maybe the relationship wasn't strong enough to hold together for the duration. I'm just not sure what the whole cause was. But, you know, this separation process was certainly an example of being normal!

For a while, I was petrified of socializing or even thinking of being with anyone. I was defensive and afraid of being rejected. I couldn't even think about meeting someone and developing a relationship. For some time, I wrestled with my turmoil. My Catch-22 was that I craved a relationship with all the goodies, but my self-image was so poor that I could not see any reason for anyone to be interested in a person who was useless.

I only felt that way every so often. It would float past me, and I would have to look back into my world and grasp my own importance. I'd have to get back on track. Every so often, I would begin to get stuck, but I'd put my blinders back on, tighten my jaw, and move forward. Soon I'd see something that would reveal what I was supposed to do.

An important component of the poststroke rebuilding process is socializing. When I was in the hospital, my family, fiancée, and close friends came to my turf; the hospital was safe. When I got together with my friends, it was a bit uncomfortable; it was not that they were uncaring, but sometimes they didn't know how to approach me. A pivotal point was the new Rod being accepted by the old friends. Not long after I'd come home from the hospital, Gary and Bill picked me up to go to a big party. As the party evolved, some of the people who didn't know me or my history looked at me as if I was weird, but most people were so positive! "Glad you're here!", "Good seeing you!", and "You're looking great!" were typical greetings. With more and more positive experiences, I began to lose some of my anxiety and fear of rejection. Both my male and female friends gave me wonderful hugs and demanded that I shake with my *right* hand.

Things were just fitting into a groove of acceptance, when all of a sudden, a beautiful woman grabbed my hand and pulled me away from the guys. She said, "Let's dance! This is my favorite song! My name is Lucy." The guys recognized my resistance to the unknown. "Yeah, Rod! Dance your feet off! Come on! You can do it! Here's your big chance! We're behind you!" I looked into Lucy's eyes and saw her support, too. My resistance dissolved, and I danced for the rest of the night! That was a great experience, and it was a good basis for my social life. At most social functions, I got all sorts of mixed messages and feelings. If I was into a male competitive situation, I felt inadequate. When I was overwhelmed by my poor self-esteem and self-image, I felt as if I was worth less than half a person! Or, if I was meeting a woman that I really wanted to develop a relationship with, I felt unable to offer what I imagined she must want! What a paradox! I was handicapping myself by limiting myself to get what I want! Or I prevented myself from taking a chance in the real world. (This mind-set kept me sputtering for about three years.)

Thinking back over this period in my life, I have come to realize that many women approached me to "check me out" and that I escaped from them, not because I wasn't interested, but because I saw myself as inadequate as a person. I sabotaged myself before they could reject me! Can you believe this? It is so self-destructive! The remarkably stupid aspect of this self-contempt is that when you get through your own baggage or garbage, you realize that the solution is so simple! No one is perfect! Everyone has their own foibles! Everyone has their handicaps; some are just more obvious than others! Everyone's limits produce other components of themselves that are much stronger! It's not the situation that is important—rather, it's what you do with it.

What a realization! Even today, I catch myself looking at the "half-empty" glass, and I have to reframe it as "half full." It took many years for me to realize that one of my behaviors during my survival mode was sabotaging my advancement. To illustrate this point, during the long survival process, it was an absolute necessity to grow my hair long and especially to take drugs. At that time, I felt that I was a victim of discrimination. I thought that I was still being teased and misunderstood. People were looking down on me and they thought poorly of me because I was "handicapped"—less than a whole person. I was one of those nonproductive, useless wastes and burdens of society. I didn't like the pain and anguish of that role. During that decade, it was "in" to have long hair and take drugs. By appearing in that role, it gave me a valid explanation and an excuse to be "different" and "spacey." The drugs offered me an excuse for my limp and for the slow, confusing nature of my verbal communication.

It eventually became clear to me that by living this way, I was handicapping myself. This deviant role was an extension of my survival needs; I had to live through the unbelievable pain. After a while, however, other aspects of my personality became stronger. I realized that drugs were now hindering my potential. It took a while because I was afraid that without the drugs I couldn't face the painful situation of being disabled. I edged into the role of being an advocate for the disabled. I was embraced by other people (both those who are disabled and those who are not) and became more self-accepting. Eventually, I was able to share my "miracles" and care for others' needs. This book is hopefully an extension of this growth in my own life.

10

Something Lost but Something Gained

When survivors confront the inevitable problems associated with recovery from a stroke, they often reveal new or rarely seen strengths that may be just as surprising to them as to others who know them well. Rod McLean found a new level of persistence and a new clarity of vision regarding his future life and career. These changes, in turn, led to a new level of commitment to education. While a stroke is never desirable, the discovery of new or buried strengths is often an unexpected benefit that makes the stroke a little easier to bear. Stroke survivors also, however, often discover certain unanticipated losses that hamper the recovery process, making it more difficult and painful.

Facing Challenges, Finding Support

The world was certainly different for Rod when he returned home. Most of the other people we interviewed similarly described the world they reentered after having their stroke as quite different from the world they had lived in previously. Shimberg (1990, p. 51) suggests that the stroke survivor's return home is particularly difficult because it conjures up so many emotions. Everyone is happy about the homecoming, yet everyone (including the survivor) is also fearful about what it will mean in terms of their role in the recovery process. Each family member is "happy that [the survivor] is leaving the hospital [or rehab center], nervous that you don't know how to care for him [or her], angry that you've been placed in this difficult position, frightened that he [or she] might have another stroke, and exhausted from lack of sleep and the tension and strain you've been under."

Each of these causes of anxiety, tension, confusion, and ambiguity for family members is amplified at least fivefold for the stroke survivors themselves. In this chapter, we will be exploring the nature of these emotional issues and the new reality that survivors and family members face. We will identify and try to understand the typical reactions of survivors when they return home and discover that they can never truly "go home again," given that they are not quite the same people that they were prior to the stroke.

New Realities

Sheila realized from the first day of awareness after her stroke that the changes she was now facing were profound. From that day forward, she progressed slowly, never feeling as though she was accomplishing anything great. Yet she knew deep within that she would someday be able to walk and talk again. She does not remember feeling like giving up. However, her son pointed out that she experienced periods of depression. Most of Sheila's friends were supportive, which enabled her to get on with her life. Progress was gradual. She might be moving slowly, but she was always moving forward.

Georgia also refused to give up. She observed that "when I reentered my 'new world,' it was difficult at first, but I knew I could fight this thing. It's funny—even at my darkest hour, I always saw light at the end of the tunnel. . . . I'm a survivor and I know it and my strength within helped me deal with my new world. It was scary, but I've hung in there and I will continue to."

Betsy was similarly impacted when she came home from the hospital. She would sometimes cry at night after her stroke, when family members were not present. She felt particularly sorry for herself when she could not do things she could do before. During her interview, Betsy repeated several times that not being able to do the same things was disgusting at first and that she would soon feel both sad and angry. She was particularly afraid of falling down stairs and still is reticent to walk up or down any steps. She is now able to navigate with the use of a cane or walker but does not use escalators or public buses because of her sense of physical vulnerability. Like many stroke survivors, she may also be reluctant to venture out into the world because she is a bit ashamed of her physical appearance and behavior in public. She feels that one of the most visible effects of the stroke is that she has to think before she talks. Betsy says that she can see the answer but it won't come out. She is aware of people noticing that she talks slowly.

Many of the people we interviewed only began to confront the fact that their world had changed when they returned home. Somehow, in the hospital and rehab center—with their intensive focus on medical treatment and rehabilitation—one can often avoid the long-term implications of disability. However, the moment the stroke survivors walk into their home and compare their status with that of just a few weeks or months before, the recognition of change sets in and the emotions begin to pour out.

Carla was one of the stroke survivors who only began to consider the implications of her stroke—and, in particular, her paralysis—when she returned home. While in the hospital, she had asked someone if she'd be able to walk again. They said perhaps, by holding on to something. At home, she realized that recovery was going to take a while, and so a nurse came for several months to help out. Carla is now in a wheelchair and has paralysis on her left side. She is able to lift her arm and move her fingers; she can lift her left leg in front of her but can't flex the ankle. She speaks with just a slight impairment and does not appear to have any trouble expressing her ideas. She says that she did not lose any of her memory or mental functions but sometimes wonders whose hand it is when she looks at her body. When she flexes her right ankle, it feels as if her left ankle is also flexing.

Carla would agree with Rod's observation that the daily struggle with gaining greater access to and control over what used to be simple bodily functions takes on major importance during the rehabilitation process. She is understandably preoccupied with these physical struggles and has little energy left for other aspects of her life. Her life is dramatically different from what it was. Like many stroke survivors, she has had to severely narrow her scope in terms of life interests and challenges. By focusing in on a few things that she can make better, Carla is able to keep a positive attitude and strong motivation to improve.

A few stroke survivors we interviewed saw the new world following their stroke as pretty much the same as the old world. This may be an accurate perception, either because their stroke was not severe or because their family and friends have done an effective job of supporting them or buffering them from a changed world. However, Tom indicated that he was respected in his community before he had his stroke but now feels isolated. Other parts of his life have changed dramatically, and he must confront these differences. Tom doesn't like to get out now because of his confinement to a wheelchair and his "memory problem": "I know what I want to say but I just can't get it out." His memory and aphasia problems bother him greatly—though when he talked about his emotions, both his memory and speech were clear.

When Beth returned home, she found that her children had completely decorated a bedroom for her on the lower floor of her house. The hospital provided a physical therapist and visiting nurse as follow-up medical services. Initially, she was given an anticoagulant drug and told not to be alone because of the danger of excessive bleeding if she fell or cut herself. Her children began taking shifts to be with her twenty-four hours a day because of this condition. Beth spoke with great appreciation of her family's support during this period. After this initial sharing of responsibility among family members, her son moved into her home and still lives there. Thus, for Beth, major changes occurred following the stroke; however, her family provided such extensive support that any fears she might have had regarding her recovery were alleviated. Beth does face a new reality but can do so without having to take many risks or rapidly learn many new survival skills. With substantial family support, she is able to gradually confront the new world she is entering and acquire the new skills she needs to live in it.

Balancing Challenge and Support

It appears that a key factor in poststroke adaptation is an appropriate balance between challenge and support. On the one hand, stroke survivors must be challenged—they must be given or allowed to assume sufficient independence to create their new selves. They must not be overprotected or stifled by patronizing attitudes and behavior—whether from well-meaning family members or from members of the medical profession. On the other hand, stroke survivors must experience sufficient and appropriate support. Family members and medical professionals must be there with physical assistance, counseling, and emotional reassurance, especially when the survivors are first recovering from the immediate physical effects of the stroke (including the impact of medication used to counteract short-term effects). When only challenge is available, stroke survivors are overwhelmed and immobilized by the impingement of uncontrollable forces. When only support is available, they are unable or unmotivated to take the often-painful steps needed toward freedom and renewal.

Beth experienced the balance between challenge and support, as did Tom and Sheila. Other stroke survivors have not been as fortunate. Frequently, vacillation occurs between too much support and too much challenge. There never seems to be an acceptable balance. Greta, for example, has found that one of the hardest things about having a stroke and suffering partial paralysis has been her loss of independence—having to depend on others for so much. For her, this involves too much support and not enough challenge. Although she appreciates all the help her friends offer—which even includes having someone cut her food while she is eating—she has been independent all her life and doesn't want to become helpless. She feels that she may not be as independent as she once was but that she doesn't have to see herself as dependent, either. Finding a new balance may be one of the most difficult aspects of recovery from a stroke for someone like her.

When the interview was over, Greta gave the interviewer a quite different sense that at other times and in other places she has inadequate support and overwhelming challenges. After the interview, Greta had to pick up her mail and asked the interviewer to accompany her. She must descend steep wooden steps out her back door to gain access to her mailbox. The top few steps have no railing. Greta had the interviewer walk ahead of her but stated that although afraid of falling, she forces herself to do this task when no one is around. For Greta, the issue of appropriate and inappropriate levels of challenge and support is critical. Should she take this risk in picking up her mail unassisted, or should she ask for help in performing this task?

What are appropriate areas in which a stroke survivor should ask for support? What are appropriate areas and to what extent should caregivers and other family members and friends offer assistance? Greta and many other stroke survivors (and caregivers) must determine the right levels of challenge and support at several points during the recovery process. More support might be needed early on, or there may be a few critical points late in the recovery process when a bit more support is needed (especially when the survivor gets discouraged or confronts unanticipated obstacles). Greta may have chosen too much challenge and insufficient support. Other stroke survivors lean too far in the other direction.

Some survivors consider their world to be unchanged following their stroke, because the new poststroke realities are too frightening or because these new realities will require substantial change in their current lives and in their hopes for the future. When asked what it was like for her when she reentered the "real world," Alice replied, "Not much different . . . same as always. The world is going faster now and it's hard to keep up." She said that she gets tired faster, so she goes to bed much earlier. For Alice and many other stroke survivors, the prospect of facing a new world is terrifying. Therefore, they must construct a world that differs very little from the one they occupied before their stroke, even if this means a major distortion of reality. In this denial, they typically hold two sets of inconsistent pictures of the world. They declare, like Alice, that nothing much has changed since their stroke, yet note that they go to bed much earlier, don't go out in public any more, or have many more fights with their husband. Somehow the individual changes are acceptable. It is not acceptable, however, to acknowledge that all of these seemingly small, isolated changes add up to a new reality and a new set of challenges for them in this poststroke world.

Feelings About and Within the New Realities

One of the effects of confronting poststroke realities is that after having strokes, people tend to experience strong feelings. Some stroke survivors, like Betsy, spoke of disgust, frustration, and anger in working with a recalcitrant body. Others reported regret and guilt regarding the part that they themselves took in setting up the conditions for their stroke. They talked about poor eating habits, preoccupation with work, unresolved and stressful relationships with family members, or failure to take care of their bodies.

After talking at some length about food and how much she missed baking and other forms of cooking, Margaret turned to what she described as personal failure on her part, both in the past and at present. She repeatedly expressed regret that "if I had taken better care of myself, I might never have had the stroke." She reported that her first poststroke doctor had reinforced this perception while encouraging her to take better care of herself today. Margaret never liked this man and shifted to a new physician. Her new doctor wants her to get more exercise. She says that her husband has been good about walking since he had his heart attack but that it is a lot harder for her: "I just slow him up."

Margaret can walk about a mile each morning; it takes her about an hour to do so. Her husband walks two and a half miles in about the same time. "I'm doing better. . . . When I first started, going to the end of the block and back was almost an all-morning affair." She laughed and then again expressed regret at not having taken better care of herself prior to her stroke. In Margaret's case, the regret about prestroke neglect of health has become a primary motivator for her to exercise, despite the fact that this exercise must initially be restricted and no doubt can be painful. For other stroke survivors, the regret and guilt associated with their stroke have led to depression and even suicidal thoughts rather than to productive life-style changes.

Other dominant poststroke feelings concern the fear and anticipation associated with the recovery process. Both Eldon and his wife were tearful and Eldon became extremely emotional when discussing his neighbor, who also recently had a stroke. This event seems to be a catalyst for Eldon's emotions. Eldon indicated that he became emotional because his neighbor was in worse shape than he. Eldon's wife, however, suggested that Eldon was anxious about his neighbor's stroke because it brought up a lot of fear regarding his own stroke. She indicated that he relived his stroke when first hearing of his neighbor's stroke. Unlike many of the other survivors we interviewed, Eldon was apparently not struck with the long-term implications of his stroke either in the hospital or when he arrived home. Rather, it took the tangible, physical evidence of another person's stroke to bring home these implications.

Eldon is highly frustrated with the body he now has to deal with and repeats this over and over again. He mentioned that one of the men in his support group had a spontaneous remission from a debilitating stroke. He insinuated that he would hope for the same thing to happen to him. He could then go on living the life to which he is accustomed. Later, Eldon's wife noted that he prays every night for full recovery and repeatedly asks her if full recovery is possible. She responds by stating that "you should count your blessings. Some people aren't doing as well as you." Thus, for Eldon, there is a volatile mixture of emotions ranging from fear to hope. He looks to both his wife and God for reassurance in dealing with these emotions and may find that his emotions are the guideposts or at least the motivators for his own recovery.

Critical Incidents and Moments of Transition

What are the turning points for people who have had strokes? What tends to bring them out of their depression, their fear, their self-doubts? As one might expect, many different kinds of critical moments were identified. Many of the people we interviewed identified family members or others as key to their poststroke achievements. Georgia credited her family and God: "My family's love and support is what pulled me out of my self-pity and gave me the strength to best this thing. They have loved and cared for me these last two years. I know if I hadn't had their love, I would have probably died in that hospital bed. Also, if God hadn't given me the inner strength I have, who knows what could have happened to me." Later she provided more detail: "When I got out of the hospital, I didn't want my family to fuss over me like a baby. I wanted to learn to do things for myself. I guess that's when my entire orientation to life changed. I soon realized that this was my new life and I better get used to it, and ever since then, I have a better and more positive outlook on my 'new life.'"

Thus, it was not her family per se that provided the impetus and the insights for Georgia. Rather, it was in reaction to her family's offers of assistance that she began to identify her need for independence and her capacity to adapt to her stroke. Undoubtedly, her family's continuing support was also critical. Georgia was fortunate, for some families are resentful when a stroke survivor asserts any independence. They conclude that the survivor isn't being appreciative of their attention or is being stubborn and resistant to rehabilitation. When this occurs, a family can set up barriers to the independence and self-esteem that most survivors need if they are going to successfully construct a new sense of self.

For some stroke survivors, the "family" they interact with at work has an even greater impact on their recovery than has their at-home family. This is to be expected; after all, many people spend more time with their colleagues at work than they do with their spouses, children, or other family members. In addition, a surprisingly large number of the stroke survivors we interviewed live alone and are estranged from or live a long distance from any family members that might have been sources of support. Sean exemplifies the independent, career-oriented stroke survivor. He attributes his turn toward rehabilitation to fellow workers and, in particular, his boss. In describing his poststroke adaptation, Sean first recalled that his initial referral for physical therapy fell through. He indicated that he was "very upset, very unhappy" to learn that the physical therapist to whom he was assigned was away for a holiday. He had already waited patiently for an opening in the rehab facility at his local hospital. Instead of giving up or simply remaining frustrated, he made use of the services of an occupational therapist and showed rapid improvement. He was diligent in performing the exercises the occupational therapist gave him, working in a focused and determined manner.

After a few weeks, Sean finally got into rehab at his hospital but was still feeling like he was doing everything himself: "I couldn't make the adjustment to asking for help . . . finally I broke down when my boss came to see me." At this point in the interview, Sean became tearful and needed to take a minute to compose himself. He had previously mentioned that he had a close working relationship with other members of his team and, in particular, with the two other men with whom he had developed a new program in Canada. Sean's stroke created a shift in the world that he inhabited with his two colleagues. He was living in a fast-moving, high-flying world of international entrepreneurship, had carefully calculated future transitions in his career, and had already been moving in an orderly, controlled fashion toward his goals. Then the stroke hit him in the midst of this high-pressure, controlled and controllable life. Somehow the appearance of his boss—as a representative of his previous life—in his new world of uncertainty and lack of control had broken through the denial Sean had erected around his impairment: "I came to realize that there was support out there." He did not have to abandon his old life and friends. They would still be there for him as he came to adjust to a slower pace and a new life-style.

As Sean continued his narrative, it became apparent that control was still a central organizing motif in his life. However, his emphasis has changed: "I used to be a go-getter. Now I concentrate on going slow and maintaining control." He seems to have developed some empathy with regard to the damaged part of himself: "It's like my right side is fifty years old and my left side is eight months old." He realizes that there is a physical imbalance, and he's able to acknowledge this new reality. Still, in his current position, Sean cannot always afford to acknowledge his new sense of vulnerability, for he is now turning his attention back to the world and a new job search.

Sometimes a medical or mental health professional, rather than a family member or colleague, provides the inspiration for stroke survivors. Bob happened to attend a conference two years after his stroke. The speaker at this meeting talked about how professionals strive too hard, lose the quality of their lives, and often destroy themselves in the process. Bob felt that the talk was directed at him. Afterward, he spoke to the presenter (a mental health professional) and made an appointment. Bob said he spent the first three sessions just crying and venting all his pent-up feelings. At the end of six months, he felt like a "whole person again." He credited the counselor with "saving my life."

Like Sean and many of the other men we interviewed, Bob had placed himself throughout his adult life in high-pressure situations; he viewed his body as essentially indestructible and saw quality of life as secondary to career accomplishments. For many men—including Sean and Bob—a stroke serves as a dramatic, unavoidable message to slow down. In many instances, however, the message is only received after the survivor gets some professional counseling or sage advice from a trusted friend or family member. While a stroke can never be denied, survivors can gradually forget the message or reinterpret it to mean that life events can't be controlled or even influenced. The finely balanced challenge and support other people offer at certain times during a stroke survivor's recovery often spell the difference between successful and unsuccessful recovery. They help the survivor turn the corner toward hopeful, proactive reconstruction of self.

Celeste identified her social worker as critical to her turnaround. Sheila similarly pointed to the assistance of her physical therapist, as well as to her son's help. Sheila asked her physical therapist what she could do about her slow progress toward verbal communication and was told that maybe she should concentrate on something else for a while— such as learning to drive again. Her son set out to teach her and within a year, she was driving on her own. With this achievement, Sheila began to regain the sense of independence that was so precious to her. She has gone on to tackle many other projects.

Spending a lot of time with her grandchildren has helped considerably. Sheila is no longer afraid to go to the zoo, get in a paddleboat, or fly to a nearby island and go sailing. She is enjoying her life and is doing so because she refuses to see anything she has done as unsuccessful. Everything learned has been a success for her, whether she has learned new skills or relearned old skills. Sheila's physical therapist taught her that the key is not to get bogged down with a barrier, but instead to shift attention to another arena in which success can be achieved. Much as Sean shifted his attention to occupational therapy when his physical therapist went on vacation, Sheila shifted her attention from speaking to physical mobility and was successful.

When Thelma was discharged from the hospital, she received an outpatient referral to a psychiatrist at a nearby clinic and had five sessions with him. She felt he was "too young" to understand anything she was saying and never trusted him: "I think he just wanted to take my money." She never confided her suicidal thoughts to him. The turnaround for Thelma began when she confided her despair to a close friend (who was a professor at a local community college) about three months after her stroke. He told her that if she killed herself she would have to wander on the earth as a ghost until her God-appointed time arrived. He also indicated that it was her God-given duty to fight to stay alive and recover. This remarkable advice served as an impetus for her rehabilitation and brought her suicidal thoughts to an end. While such advice may not be appropriate for all stroke survivors who are depressed, it certainly had an effect on Thelma!

Many other survivors pointed to newfound friends as sources of their turnaround—particularly within stroke clubs and other self-help groups. Eldon feels that he received excellent care through his hospital and physician. The ongoing exercise classes offered by the local community center were very helpful. The most valuable resource, however, has been the local stroke support group that he regularly attends with his wife. They both think that it was and still is very important for them to attend, since they are able to interact with others who have experienced the same trauma. They feel that without this assistance, they would have a pervasive sense of helplessness and overwhelming fear. With the lectures and other activities provided by the support group, they are more in touch with and prepared to deal with changes in their life-style and relationship. They also find that the support group is a source of new friends who have experienced similar life events and are coping with similar problems. This friendship function is particularly valuable if the stroke survivor no longer has a spouse or close family members to rely on for support and companionship.

Some of the people we interviewed said that there were no distinct turning points for them—much as some of the people we interviewed said that the world had not changed dramatically for them after they had their stroke. Alice said that she can't remember any turning points per se when she began to move forward. She said that she never felt like giving up—that she always felt that if she worked enough, she would get better. Alice indicated that the exercises she performs help her progress and that she has gone everywhere she could to exercise or work in a heated pool. No person or thing in particular stands out for her as an impetus for her to begin this work after her stroke.

Other stroke survivors who reported no turning point certainly seem to be in need of such an event or person. Tom stated that he has tried to get help from other people by attending several different stroke clubs. However, in each case, he became bored and concluded that it wasn't worth the effort. When he first arrived home, a visiting nurse came in twice a week to bathe him, but now she only comes once a week, because—once again—it's too much trouble for him. Tom isn't interested in getting out and would rather just stay home. He appears to be unwilling to confront all of the challenges associated with movement into the outside world. Most stroke survivors must deal with the stares of strangers, the ill-timed offers of assistance by well-intentioned but insensitive friends and strangers, and the embarrassment of slow physical motion and halting speech. Tom found no gratification in the stroke clubs he attended; hence there was no need to confront these challenges. As we noted previously, adaptation to strokes requires a balance between challenge and support. Tom was unable to find any satisfactory support (other than his long-suffering wife), hence was unwilling to take on any challenges. He remains at home, finding little to excite or test him as well as little to console or teach him with regard to the processes of renewal.

Tom's story is particularly sad, because his first wife died of a lingering illness and his second wife's first husband had also been an invalid for a number of years before he died. Tom and Effie (his wife) had planned to travel, but with a severe accident experienced by his son and Tom's own stroke, "that all went down the river." Tom now feels stuck in one place, and nothing has occurred to provide an impetus for any shift in this position. One can anticipate that without this impetus, Tom will become yet another invalid for his second wife. We can expect her to take care of Tom but to grow more resentful about his own inaction and the unfair burden placed on her by fate or by her selection of husbands.

What advice might we give Tom and other stroke survivors like him who seem to be stuck in their rehabilitation efforts? To reiterate, the answer appears to reside at least in part in the balance between challenge and support. If Tom was encouraged to get a bit more support for himself (rather than relying exclusively on his wife), maybe he would be willing to take on more challenges and continue his rehabilitation. Other stroke survivors might wish to begin from the opposite direction, by being encouraged or allowed to seek a little more challenge through increased independence. Then, paradoxically, the support that other people wish to offer will become more acceptable, for there is now more need for this support. Such is the way of challenge and support. They tend to work as two sides of the rehabilitation coin. When there is more of one, there is an increased need for the other.

What strengths do successful survivors possess, and what gains do they identify in making sense of their new poststroke life? Conversely, what are the losses that stroke survivors experience and how do they come to terms with the grieving associated with these losses? We turn now to each of these considerations.

Personal Strengths and Unanticipated Gains

Typically, one cannot readily predict whether a stroke survivor is likely to gain from this massive life intrusion or to succumb to the negative and often permanently debilitating effects of the stroke. Attitude seems to be critical. On the one hand, survivors may have much to live for but may choose to let the stroke defeat them. James came to a local rehabilitation center from another state, having moved to live with his daughter. He had held an executive position in a large corporation; he was highly intelligent and had obviously been a very competent businessperson. But his stroke left him quite aphasic. He had suffered depression in the past when his wife died and was now suffering from the loss of his former self, his loss of communication, and the loss of his job.

James entered speech and physical therapy and was soon able to walk again and used a cane to move easily from place to place. His communication skills, however, were only progressing slowly. He was a proud man and found it frustrating to be unable to express himself. Unfortunately, in some instances, pride is based on or leads to avoidance rather than perseverance. James briefly saw a psychiatrist who put him on an antidepressant drug, which helped for a while. He still becomes frustrated with his lack of communication, however, and this frustration seems to have hindered his rehabilitation efforts rather than serving as an incentive (as in the case of Rod). He went to a few sessions of a stroke support group, where he expressed himself slightly but not the way he wanted to be heard. As a result, he rarely tried to speak and eventually dropped out of the group.

James certainly has reason to be discouraged and depressed. He has lost both his wife and his career. Yet he also has much to be thankful for: a supportive daughter, physical mobility, continuing use of his intellectual gifts, and financial security. As Rod suggested, stroke survivors may choose to see the glass as half empty or half full. They must make this choice, which will impact their entire rehabilitation effort. So far, James has tended to be pessimistic.

By contrast, we can look to the attitude of Jessie, a woman who is over seventy-five years old and, like James, highly intelligent. Jessie also lost her husband several years ago, having cared for him for many years prior to his death. She fell down when she had her stroke and still has a balance problem. Unlike James, Jessie has trouble getting around. She is also unable to focus and read the way she did before her stroke, so that she is at a much greater disadvantage than James with regard to the use of her intellect. Initially, Jessie was determined to stay in her home of fifty years. Her daughter, who lives in another state, wanted her to move in with her, but Jessie refused. She now lives in her own home with the help of neighbors. She shares her story with many people in the group, who are amazed to hear of her determination and perseverance. Jessie is determined to live life to the fullest. She even passed her driver's license test and drives to her support group.

Jessie is truly an amazing woman. She has the determination to make the best of what she has left in her life and finds fulfillment in life itself. For her, the glass is always at least half full. Actually, it is often overflowing! In contrast with James, who could not accept his losses, Jessie will survive and have a high-quality life. James will no doubt have an adequate and secure life; however, he may never let go of his anger and despair in order to accept and live with his limitations and celebrate the resources and skills that he still has. He simply is unable to accept himself as he now is. James and Jessie are two people of great value and potential, but only one of them can see this value and potential, can accept themselves as they are, and can build a new life.

What seem to be the positive outcomes of having a stroke, given that some survivors, like Jessie, are able to reframe their rehabilitation as an opportunity or even a gift? The major gains that stroke survivors identified during their interviews included a new sense of meaning in life, patience, interpersonal sensitivity, personal insight, spirituality, and an opportunity for change. We found repeatedly in our interviews that stroke survivors are often inclined to view their survival as not just an opportunity to discover patience or other inner strengths, but as somehow a sign of some much grander—even divine—purpose for their life. In this way, many survivors were able to find meaning in the stroke and to use their religious beliefs or spirituality as a newly awakened or reaffirmed strength.

Even for survivors who are not particularly religious, the experience of a massive life intrusion such as a stroke can lead to an alternative perspective. Sean spoke of a strength within himself—the capacity to clearly and accurately evaluate himself—yet looks outside himself for a sense of purpose. He said that his stroke has helped him appreciate the support he has received from his friends as well as from health care workers. Sean experiences a sense of purpose and value in helping others who have suffered strokes and has become more compassionate in general. The stroke has forced him to recognize his interdependence with others; he has come to realize that he needs other people and they need him.

Like many men, Sean admits that he "may have been shutting people out" earlier in his life. Other men, however, have not been as "fortunate" as Sean, for he believes that the stroke has brought him to his senses and that he can now fully appreciate other people before it's too late. One of the most intriguing findings from our study is this increasing interpersonal sensitivity to be found, in particular, among men who have had strokes. Something about the stroke has led some survivors to gain much more sensitivity to the feelings and needs of other people. Survivors also described themselves as being more attuned to lying and deception on the part of others. Sheila, for instance, believes that she is now able to determine when people are being overly "sweet" and are generally not being honest about their feelings. Thelma also reported that she has a heightened sensitivity to the unexpressed feelings of others, although (like most stroke survivors) she can't explain "how I do this." She believes that she can always tell when other people are lying "by the way they look"—a capacity she did not have before her stroke.

This newfound strength for many stroke survivors might be explained in several different ways. Perhaps in losing some verbal skills, survivors become more sensitive to nonverbal communication. Alternatively, survivors may be picking up more information about other people than they did prior to their stroke because they have to attend more closely to these other people, given their cognitive impairment. The increased sensitivity might also relate to the increased emotionality often found among stroke survivors. In gaining greater access to their own feelings, stroke survivors (and, in particular, men) may also be gaining greater access to the feelings of others.

Sheila spoke about the patience she has discovered as a personal strength since she began the process of recovery. This attribute is something new for her, and she is proud of having acquired it. She also takes great pride in having learned the skill of making decorative sugar eggs. Both big and small accomplishments are important to her—and to most other stroke survivors. Just as these men and women must plan for and take small steps on the way to overcoming large, long-term obstacles, they also are inclined to take pleasure and pride in both small and large accomplishments.

Sheila has been able to slowly gain power physically and interpersonally by increasing her self-esteem. She has empowered herself by becoming more independent. Physically, she has increased the strength of her left hand to the point that it is now better than her nondominant right hand was before she had her stroke. In the area of interpersonal relationships, her friends report that Sheila has been able to reestablish the same sensitivity, compassion, and directness as before the stroke. She maintains her self-confidence by completing tasks regardless of how long it may take. For example, she will complete an entire dinner by herself, including the shopping. Because she cannot write, she has discovered that if she takes the recipes with her when she is shopping, she can purchase all the necessary ingredients. It increases her self-esteem to work things out by herself. The way she maintains control over her life is by making dinner from start to finish, by driving, traveling by airplane, and, most important, living on her own.

Kari agreed with Sheila in identifying patience as the primary strength she has discovered in herself following her stroke. Kari described herself before the stroke (which occurred seven years ago) as both flighty and stubborn: "You had to hit me over the head." She had no patience with herself or other people: "I was always kind of a gadabout. I'm still out there a bit, but, I don't know, I think what I'm learning and what I have learned from having had the stroke is patience with myself and other people." With this patience, Kari can also experience forgiveness. When asked how she sees herself now as opposed to before the stroke, she replied, "It's not something that I've sat down and done—said 'here's what I was and here's what I am now.' Yes, I was a pretty fast mover and I always used to push, push, push. I don't do that quite as much now. I think I'm learning, what with the patience and the enjoyment of others, to find it easier to see what is the next step to take."

Like Sheila and Kari, Georgia looks on the stroke experience as having taught her more about herself—which came as a pleasant surprise: "I think my primary strengths now are my 'inner strengths.' I have so much determination now—more than I ever did in my life. I feel so different about life and people. It seems to me, I appreciate life a little more since I was so close to losing mine." She went on to indicate that she now listens more attentively to other people (in part because of her cognitive impairments) and even communicates with others better (once again, in compensation for her speech impairments). She indicates that she is now more inclined to express her feelings, her stroke group having been helpful in this regard: "I attend a stroke survivors' group. This has helped me a lot. Being with and talking to others like myself has given me a sense of power or strength to help myself and also help others."

Dorothy reiterated Georgia's conclusion that her poststroke recovery has been a renewing experience—particularly with regard to interpersonal relationships. She feels like a new person and does not experience the same fear of death as before her stroke. Also, she indicated that she experiences a more personal and special closeness to God. She pointed out that since her stroke, she has been more likely to see the good in people and not concentrate on the bad. She has had a real softening toward her mother. She and her mother had a difficult relationship. Her mother had been dead for several years; however, through the experience of the stroke, Dorothy has reconnected with her and believes her mother is watching out for her.

While Georgia and Dorothy have been reminded of the importance of relationships, developed determination, and found a new appreciation for life, other survivors have discovered impatience and new insights into the less favorable aspects of their lives and their own failings. They tolerated damaging conditions in their lives prior to their stroke but have wisely chosen not to tolerate these conditions any longer. The major strength these stroke survivors have discovered in themselves relates not to their increasing sensitivity to interpersonal relationships, but rather has involved confronting an existing relationship that is unsatisfactory.

Susan found herself feeling slow and helpless during the early period of her recovery. She was depressed and occasionally thought about suicide: "The depression was not from my stroke but from the way my husband was treating me. I didn't have time to think about my condition. I was too concerned about pleasing my husband." As far as he was concerned, "I was useless to him." As her husband's abuse accelerated, Susan realized that she would have to make some major changes. She began reflecting on her past actions, beliefs, and attitudes, and learned that she had played an instrumental part in the creation of a destructive marriage by colluding in her husband's abuse.

After a particularly abusive episode, Susan thought that her life was at risk. At that moment, she decided to move out and file for divorce. She also sold her large house and moved into a mobile home. She has learned that "living alone doesn't mean that I have to be lonely." Like Sheila, Susan has discovered her capacity to be autonomous. She is a strong person who does not have to be unconditionally dependent on another person. She might never have learned about her strength if the stroke had not occurred.

At this point in her life, Susan doesn't feel like a new person. However, the interviewer had known her prior to her stroke and indicated that she was in fact significantly different than before. Prior to the stroke, Susan had low self-esteem and a poor sense of self-worth. She seemed to have a fatalistic view of life. Now, she appears to be stronger and happier. She is content with her life and is "not angry anymore." She has taken major strides in dealing with her disability. She has virtually a new life as a single person and admits to enjoying the new world forced on her by the stroke. Susan does not miss the abilities that she lost after her stroke, nor the material things that she lost after the divorce: "I believe that as we grow older, we need less space and less of the material things. Who has the energy for it?"

When asked what her greatest strength was, she replied, "I believe in God. Although I am not a churchgoer, I do believe in prayer. I believe that God saved me from experiencing the actual stroke. My being unconscious during the actual event was a blessing from God. A person can only take so much." Many of the stroke survivors, like Susan, have looked to their religious beliefs or some other aspect of spirituality for strength following the stroke. Though the stroke could be viewed as a sign that God doesn't really care about a person's welfare or that a benevolent God doesn't exist, most survivors interpreted their survival as a sign of God's existence and grace. In some cases, stroke survivors—like Susan—felt they were spared pain during their stroke because God was watching over them.

Many other survivors also draw great strength from their continuing faith. Betsy feels that her faith has been the cornerstone of her ability to cope with her stroke, her new life, and her feelings about both. Although she experienced some sadness and anger following the stroke, she has never felt like giving up. Betsy usually draws on her faith when she is feeling down and tries to maintain a positive attitude.

Eldon believes that his spirituality and that of his wife were a major strength for him during recovery. He mentioned that even his physician provided spiritual support. Eldon became emotional when describing the support he has received from his family and friends. The spiritual strength he has experienced seems to be intimately linked with the more secular support and strength he receives from other people. Eldon still asks "Why me?" but is more concerned with getting back to the "old me." He wants to return to the busy life-style he once enjoyed with his work, family, and friends.

Kari also talked about spirituality when describing her poststroke strengths. Her eyes filled with tears as she spoke of her spiritual relationship with God: "It is becoming, and is, very important in my life." She fundamentally believes that her stroke was in fact part of a spiritual covenant: "I honestly think that I had been trying to learn these lessons [about patience] earlier, or somehow my body or my life was trying to help me—help point out what I needed to do to continue working on the things that needed changing. I think that's what life is about anyhow—about change and learning to accept and being willing to accept it. I somehow have the feeling that I decided that I would be willing to do it this way, if I didn't learn it earlier with the previous attempts in my life."

Thus, Kari preserved her religious beliefs while confronting the intrusion of a major medical problem. She decided that the stroke was a message to her about patience and the meaning of life that she, as a stubborn and driven person, wasn't open to learning previously. Many stroke survivors spoke of their prestroke resistance to important priorities and values and of the extent to which the stroke forced them to reexamine and reassess these priorities and values.

For those stroke survivors—like Thelma—who did at least temporarily lose their faith in God following the stroke, poststroke recovery was particularly difficult emotionally and physically. Thelma became increasingly despondent and suicidal. She felt abandoned by God and by other people. She thought no one in her family really cared about her or was even aware of how she felt. Perhaps she felt abandoned by God precisely because of her sense that everyone else in her life had also abandoned her. Our religious beliefs can often be comforting even when others are not there for us. However, as we observed with regard to Eldon, we often find God more easily when we also feel loved and supported by those who are closest to us and most dear.

Religious faith has certainly been a major strength for many survivors. These men and women have stepped back into a world that is dramatically different from what it was prior to the intrusion of the stroke. Continuity in religious belief can provide the bridge between the old and new realities, as well as the context for finding meaning in this seemingly arbitrary and destructive life event. The bridge provided by religion is often particularly important for stroke survivors who come from traditional cultures with strong religious roots. Zelman (1992) points out that many of the African American survivors she has studied believe that there has been divine intervention in their recovery. Given that the church plays such an important role in the lives of many of the African Americans Zelman sees, it is not surprising that religion is such a source of comfort and continuity.

One of the men we interviewed, John, declared that his entire world was turned upside down and now he is left picking up the pieces. He admits that this process has not been easy, but it has opened his eyes to a few things—much as Susan's stroke opened her eyes to the true nature of her destructive marriage and Sean's stroke opened his eyes to the value of his relationships with others. John's eye-opening experience, however, was dramatically different from those of Susan and

Sean. In particular, his relationships with his God and with those he once considered friends have changed. As we noted in Chapter Eight, John's identity had been wrapped up around his church and the many friends with whom he socialized. Now he does not attend church and spends most of his days alone. Unfortunately, for him, the stroke experience exacerbated the tendency to be self-sufficient (a tendency he shares with many men).

While newfound strengths have led to new lives and enhanced self-esteem for both Sheila and Susan, John has experienced partial stagnation and withdrawal. He would benefit from a new appreciation of the complexity of human relationships. After the stroke, he naively relied on members of his church for support and understanding, without realizing that his relationships with them must change in order for them to be helpful to him. Both he and they must change a bit, given his new, poststroke world. John was apparently unwilling to make these changes. He failed to discover the patience that Sheila found or perhaps the strength associated with flexibility and empathic understanding of other people's fears and needs that became evident to Kari following her stroke.

But John has some newly discovered strengths. First, he did not lose his faith in God. Rather, like Susan, he reconceived this faith in a new, inspirational manner. He firmly believes that he was spared death because something is in store for him on earth. He feels that his mission is not complete and strives to fulfill the wishes of this higher power. While he does not yet know what his mission is, he is attuned to new purposes and meaning in his life, which keeps him from becoming too stagnant in his isolated life-style.

While John is stepping back into a world with many fewer friends, he views this experience as a process of becoming authentic. He can now more clearly see himself and his own strengths and limitations and can also more clearly see the hypocrisy in other people. At this stage in his life, he is not invested in pleasing others. Rather, he is focusing his energies on developing a truly authentic relationship with those close to him. Like many others, John has tended to have fewer friends as he has grown older. However, one wonders how he will be able to sustain the few critical relationships he has if he does not discover the complementary strengths of tolerance and forgiveness.

John must recognize his own hypocrisy and his own desire to hide behind false or superficial aspects of his public self. In recovering from a stroke, one is in an excellent position to learn about fear, self-doubt, and the desire to hide. Many of the people we interviewed spoke of such insights about themselves and others. Hopefully, John will learn about this, too—perhaps before he discovers and embarks on his life mission.

Like many others we interviewed, John was fortunate in having prestroke aspects of his life that he could turn to during the period of recovery. Stroke survivors often return to long-term religious beliefs as a source of continuity with their previous lives. This sense of continuity is often critical to successful recovery. Even if the spiritual or other strengths that a stroke survivor identifies are newly discovered, these strengths often build on a previous coping experience that was successful and that is still fresh in the survivor's mind.

Alice, for example, spoke about "self-determination" when asked to identify a primary, poststroke strength. She referred back to a previous experience, however, in first discussing this strength: "When I came to this country, I did not speak English and I figured it wouldn't be easy. So I took courses at the university and learned English. It is the same thing now." While John and Susan could return to earlier experiences in their lives where faith in God was justified as a way of keeping up their "God-given strength" during the stroke recovery process, Alice relied on strengths that she knew were there at a previous point in her life—when learning how to speak English.

While continuity was a source of strength for many stroke survivors, discontinuity provided strength for other survivors. In many instances, survivors identified their major poststroke strength as their capacity to stop doing something unhealthy that they did prior to their stroke. Susan found the resolve and courage to break away from her abusive husband and obtain a divorce. Bob quit being a "work machine" as a result of his stroke and now finds that his life has more quality and enjoyment. Since his stroke, Bob sold his business and now works two days per week in another business as an employee. He says that he can work more slowly and sells fewer products. He plans to retire within two years.

Greta similarly believes that her previous life-style, which included social drinking, smoking, and eating rich foods, contributed to her stroke. She has made dramatic life-style changes as a result of becoming involved with holistic medicine and is almost entirely a vegetarian. She no longer smokes or drinks and is amazed at how much better she feels physically as a result of her dietary changes. "I don't want to say, if only I had done this, then this wouldn't have happened to me." However, she does consider this new life-style and her commitment to holistic medicine a newfound strength associated with the loss of prestroke life-style choices.

The most positive change for Carla since her stroke has been her cessation of drinking. She states that she "dare not" drink now. While she believes that the stroke could have been related to her drinking, she doubts this causal connection. Nevertheless, the stroke led her to a dramatic reconsideration of her life-style and priorities. She indicated during her interview that she was always able to function adequately and fulfill her responsibilities as a housewife before her stroke but felt that she wasn't very happy then and needed to drink to escape a sense of low self-esteem: "I felt like I was nobody. I wasn't something, only a mom, only a housewife."

Since her stroke, Carla has developed a better sense of herself as a person who can overcome adversity and can control her own destiny. She has dramatically demonstrated her own strength and perseverance to herself and can credit herself with keeping herself alive. She no longer needs to drink as a way of defending against her despair and sense of powerlessness. Carla stressed several times during her interview that she could easily have developed a "poor-me" attitude following her stroke. While she does mourn the losses that she has experienced as a result of the stroke, she is actively involved in her own recovery and refuses to feel sorry for herself. She attends physical therapy four times a week and participates in a local stroke club. This has improved her feelings about herself: "When I'm with people, I am a person." When she was forced to leave behind her prestroke identity and begin the rehabilitation process, Carla found purpose for the first time in her life and gained a new identity as a courageous, hard-working survivor.

Her goals for the future are to be able to walk and go to the bathroom alone. She wants to do more work in assisting other disabled people and has been thinking a lot about plans for a program in which disabled people can live in their own apartments, yet have instant access to those who can help them if needed. She is thinking about how she could take care of herself if something happened to her husband. She recently talked to a woman who is ninety and still active and indicated that this woman might be a good role model for her. Ironically, this highly active, thoughtful woman might never have existed if it was not for the self-defining event of the stroke. This intrusive event has given Carla a focal point for her diffuse energy. She no longer has to define herself—as do many women her age—solely with reference to other people (as a "wife," "homemaker," or "mother") but can speak of herself as a "stroke survivor." She can direct attention not only to her own recovery, but also to the recovery of others with disabilities. She can look to a new role model of independence in preparing for her own years as an older adult.

Greta, Carla, and Bob have apparently not needed a sense of continuity to sustain them through their recovery. Rather, for the three of them, their old life got them into trouble and was probably not very satisfying anyway. They have discovered new strengths as a result of their stroke and now sense that life has begun anew to sustain them in their recovery efforts. Some stroke survivors find the strength of patience or determination; others find their capacity to live alone; still others find a new appreciation for life, a renewed commitment to God, or a new, life-enhancing outlook. For those who have never discovered or rediscovered these strengths, there is only stagnation during the recovery process, for, as we will document in the next section, such strengths are needed to counteract and overcome the profound losses that also are discovered during the recovery process.

Personal Limitations and Unanticipated Losses

Stroke survivors experience many losses that they had not initially anticipated or at least did not think would be a source of such difficulty—ranging from the loss of physical mobility to the loss of a job to the loss of friends. Mary typifies many stroke survivors, especially those with relatively severe impairments. Her social worker reported that she became a different person after her stroke. She suffers from noticeable confusion and memory impairment. When taken shopping, she becomes confused, cannot pick out her size, and usually wanders aimlessly around the clothing racks. She frequently mispronounces or substitutes wrong words while speaking. Like many stroke survivors, Mary must confront on a daily basis a series of small losses, each of which compounds the problem of retaining or rebuilding a sense of self-esteem and self-sufficiency. Every time she tries to return to her old life—such as shopping for clothes—she is reminded of her limitations and often ends the day, as her social worker observed, "staring helplessly" at her radically changed world.

Many other stroke survivors similarly spoke of their loss of cognitive or communication abilities. Todd initially lost his ability to read but has been able to recover this skill. He continues to improve, and a tutor meets with him weekly. Todd claims that the tutor has helped him greatly, just by bringing him books and listening to him read. As a teacher and lover of books, Todd obviously feels this particular loss deeply. The patience and understanding of his tutor have been invaluable.

The loss of certain other physical and mental functions were also often mentioned—inability to play particular sports, type or handwrite letters, sew or cut a board. These all impact on centrally valued aspects of the survivors' lives. The loss of sexual potency was also difficult for some survivors to cope with, though many of those interviewed addressed this issue with some reluctance—which is understandable. Several of the men we interviewed hesitantly talked about their fears about impotence. These fears have often been realized. In some instances, the impotence has been at least partially compensated for with a rich fantasy life; in other cases, survivors have blocked this part of their life off and deny that it is of importance any more. All too often, impotence is not caused by the stroke per se, but rather by the way survivors perceive the impact of the stroke on their sexuality.

Many of the women we interviewed either were too embarrassed to talk about their own sexuality or found it too painful to discuss their sexual losses. Thelma differed from many of her female colleagues in being able to both laugh a bit about sexuality and acknowledge her loss: "Sex is one of my fondest memories." Having been in an abusive relationship for many years, Thelma hadn't been sexually active for some time. Thus, the stroke made little difference in her own life. Sheila indicated that her first poststroke sexual experience brought on feelings of uncertainty because she was not sure how to make love. During this first sexual experience, however, Sheila derived the same amount of pleasure as she did prior to her stroke. She does not feel that the stroke has changed her identity as a sexual person. In fact, when asked whether she had had any "performance anxiety," she emphatically responded, "Are you kidding? No!" She still sees herself as a person— hence she is still sexual.

Other stroke survivors mentioned their loss of status, vocation, or a familiar life-style as particularly difficult to confront. Roberta stated that one of the difficult things for her to handle was being designated as disabled and being unable to perform her previous work duties. She had been employed during most of her adult life and felt uncomfortable not working. Like many stroke survivors who had worked all their lives or had taken great pride in their role as parent, spouse, or homemaker, Roberta felt a loss of her own identity and sense of self-worth. Initially, she was reluctant to engage in many outside activities, but eventually she found other areas of interest and importance.

She has become active in a local stroke club that meets twice a week. This support group has helped her develop a more positive attitude. The group also serves as a social group; its members go out to eat together once a month as well as participating in various other social events. Roberta indicated that some of the members are still confined to wheelchairs, but they need not feel alone or helpless. Roberta herself doesn't have to feel embarrassed about her own disabilities, since the other members of the stroke club are confronting similar problems. She has remained active in the club, and a few years ago, she escorted members on a safari in Africa. She indicated that sometimes she also helps conduct seminars for survivors and their families.

Other stroke survivors identified interpersonal losses as being particularly painful. We have already discussed John's sense of betrayal by his former friends and fellow church members. Bob similarly regrets the loss of friends and family, though he attributes this loss not to the indifference of other people, but rather to his own insensitivity: "I wasn't a nice person to be around. I hope they understand." Bob never felt that he could communicate with members of his family about his stroke or about his self-anger. Now things have improved, and Bob says he doesn't think about his stroke or that period in his life very often. He states that things are going well and he feels happy.

The interviewer, who had known Bob for eight years, offers a similar picture of the losses (and gains) that Bob has experienced. She could see changes in him that he didn't mention. Bob looks the same, and his physical disability is unnoticeable. However, he cries more easily and is otherwise more emotional than before. The interviewer remembers him as fast talking, fast living, and always in charge. He now appears—like many of the poststroke men we interviewed—to be more sensitive and easy to be around. Bob expressed discomfort with his new-found emotionality but commented that he is now more of a "total human being." He no longer has to sacrifice his humanity to retain "control" of his emotions.

Bob ended the interview—as did many stroke survivors—by saying, "Something positive has come out of this!" Thus, even with the considerable losses that survivors confront, those who have successfully recovered have gained much from the traumatic experience. They have discovered new strengths, made life-style changes, and renewed or further strengthened old commitments to family, friends, and God. Perhaps most important, they have profited from new learning with regard to themselves, other people, and life-style and other priorities.

11

Insights from
Survivors

Stroke survivors were asked to identify the major lessons they had learned while recovering from this massive life intrusion. For a successful recovery, six elements seem to be crucial: (1) control over and participation in multiple treatment plans, (2) a new perspective on life, (3) a sense of self-worth and perseverance, (4) patience, (5) the right balance between challenge and support, and (6) support from other people.

Control Over and Participation in Multiple Treatment Plans

According to John, the most important lesson to be learned from his stroke experience is that obtaining correct medical treatment is critical to successful recovery. He believes that doctors should be questioned and challenged throughout the process. John noted that many stroke survivors tend to hold doctors in such high esteem that they never question their decisions. This, according to him, is their first mistake. Many other stroke survivors similarly learned how important it is to participate actively in the formulation of their own treatment plan. Even if they trust their doctor's competence and knowledge, they still feel that in certain areas they are the most knowledgeable person around. No one knows more than the stroke survivor about energy level, physical competence, and emotional life. The recommendations of the doctors must be considered in light of these more personal insights.

175

In her words and even more in her actions, Kari points, like John, to the importance of taking control of your own treatment plan and illustrates the importance of participating in a variety of programs. During her interview, Kari mentioned physical therapy, adaptive physical education classes, psychotherapy, body therapy, an interactive physician, two support groups, and more. She has access to all these treatment programs in part because she has money. However, she also uses many low-cost or free services. When asked for suggestions on care for new stroke survivors, she mentioned peer counseling: "What we tried to do was to go and talk to people who have recently had strokes, so that we can encourage them and tell them to just go ahead and take a chance. Learn to be vulnerable; boy, am I still learning to do that!"

In the latter statement, Kari may have touched on a central factor in the use or nonuse of appropriate treatment programs. To take advantage of these programs, survivors must acknowledge that they need help and can't complete their recovery on their own. This inevitably makes people more vulnerable, for they have to rely on the expertise and support of other people. For some stroke survivors, this is hard. Their isolation and stubbornness may have even contributed to their stroke in the first place.

Yet both John and Kari spoke to the opposite issue as well. Stroke survivors should allow themselves to become vulnerable and rely on the assistance of other people only up to a point; they must also assume control over their overall treatment plan. They should not let themselves depend too much on the expertise or goodwill of others, for health professionals and family members ultimately do not know as well as the stroke survivors what is good for them. Thus, the message from both John and Kari seems to be: control your overall treatment plan, but allow others to be of assistance in the implementation of specific components of the plan.

Often at the heart of the problem of control over a treatment plan is the absence of information about appropriate and available programs. Martin, a physician who had had a stroke, spoke with passion about the need for stroke survivors to receive accurate and useful information about treatment programs. Ester confirmed Martin's point. She received no information about alternative treatment programs and believes that this is the most important lesson to be learned: find out about the resources available in your community. Bob similarly mentioned that he wished he had known about psychological support services when he was leaving the hospital, and Betsy indicated that one of the most important services she now provides to stroke survivors is information about (as well as transportation to) various treatment programs.

Shimberg (1990) recommends that stroke survivors and family members acquire as much information as possible, both immediately after the stroke and throughout the recovery process. Furthermore, she recommends that a family member take careful notes when meeting with the doctor, nurse, or rehabilitation counselor. As she notes, the information is often complex, everyone is unnerved and unfocused, and we tend to insert our own biases and assumptions about strokes when recalling what an expert has said. We would add that the task of note taker and keeper of the records can help at least one family member feel like they are making a tangible contribution to the recovery process.

A New Perspective on Life

While John emphasized the need for control over one's physical treatment, he also focused on a more psychological dimension. One of the most important things he has learned from the stroke experience is that good can result from adversity—this despite the fact that he feels profoundly let down by his friends and members of his church. John believes that he has a view of life and love that he did not possess prior to the stroke. He is much more content with himself now.

The message Roberta perceives is a little different. Yes, a stroke can produce unanticipated results; however, the most important lesson to be learned from a stroke, according to Roberta, is that the stroke itself is unanticipated. In other words, we should be prepared for unexpected traumas in our lives—what in this book we have called *intrusive life events*. Roberta has authorized someone to have power of attorney in case something similar happens to her again. She has also joined a home care service, so that emergency services can be made available to her, and now wears an identity bracelet. As further preparation for unexpected events, she has made arrangements for her cats to be taken care of if she is hospitalized or becomes incapacitated.

While these preparatory acts may be wise—especially for someone like Roberta, who lives alone—one wonders if she is too concerned with reducing the impact of future strokes or related events and not sufficiently concerned with preventing another stroke (by taking better care of herself, physically and psychologically). Fortunately, Roberta also identified a second lesson. She has learned to laugh more rather than cry. She claimed that for the first six months after her stroke, she spent most of her time crying. She has since become less interested in being a perfectionist and has learned how to slow down. She said that because of her speech difficulties, she has learned how to talk more slowly, which has helped her to be more patient and more relaxed. Perhaps, as in John's case, her most important lesson—to slow down a bit—was an unanticipated benefit of having a stroke.

A Sense of Self-Worth and Perseverance

In reflecting back on her stroke experience, Thelma mentioned that the first thing she had to fight was fear. She was afraid to go to sleep for many months, worrying that she might have another stroke in her sleep. She was afraid to be alone, because she thought she might have the stroke with no one around to help her (having recently left her abusive husband). The lesson Thelma learned concerns the way she confronted this fear—specifically the actions she took to become more self-reliant. She became determined to do everything in her power to recover and to depend on others for help as little as possible. This certainly seems appropriate for her, given the absence of much support from either her husband or her children.

Thelma does not believe that her stroke had any meaning or purpose. She believes its causes were entirely physical (age in combination with a high-cholesterol diet). Her advice to stroke survivors is to "pray a lot, exercise as much as you can, and don't wait for others to do for you. Do as much for yourself as you can." These do not seem to be idle words, for Thelma expects little from others but would like people to "care about me. And the best way to show it is just to sit and talk once in a while."

The key message from Georgia was much like Thelma's. She emphasized reaffirmation of her self-worth: "I'm not a bedridden vegetable. I am talking, breathing, feeling, and soon will be walking, and these are major successes for me as of today." Georgia said that she would tell other people like herself that they should "never give up, because once you give up on yourself, you die inside. There's always some hope at the end of the tunnel—you have to believe that." She also indicated that she thinks stroke survivors need considerable support and should never be ashamed to accept this support: "Never reject it. It makes this hell a little easier to adapt to. Believe in yourself—this is so important."

Likewise, Greta offered an inspirational message for other survivors. She welcomes the opportunity to help anyone who is dealing with a similar struggle and wants to tell other survivors to "continue to believe in yourself." Greta's courage and fighting spirit are readily apparent and have obviously contributed to her progress and successful adaptation. She summed up her philosophy as follows: "Don't assume you can't." She is a woman who truly believes in herself and assumes that she can.

Patience

Like many women we interviewed, Alice spoke of her capacity to overcome adversity as the central lesson to be learned from her stroke experience. She indicated that she would like to tell other survivors that the best way to overcome a stroke is by positive thinking. Like Georgia, Alice urged survivors to push beyond their negative thoughts: "A stroke is a temporary thing . . . it is up to the person to get rid of it as soon as possible." In the case of both Alice and Georgia, one wonders to what extent they are advocating denial and the avoidance of a realistic appraisal of their new reality. Yet for each of these remarkable women— for Alice in particular—this selective denial seems to have worked. Alice has persisted in her recovery because she refused to become depressed and because she set short-term, realistic goals. Though she did not specifically mention it, the most important lesson for her may have been patience in the accomplishment of short-term goals while overcoming her stroke-induced disabilities.

By breaking up her challenges into small, manageable units, Alice has been able to persevere. She said that some of her successes since the stroke have been modest—such as being able to make her bed every morning, fluffing her pillow, and helping her husband with the cooking. She is about to start typing again, as well as starting to write (by holding her hand so that it stays straight while she moves the pen). Alice clearly is unwilling to give up. She will not allow herself to feel defeated and is able to preserve her strong willpower by acknowledging and celebrating her own small achievements.

Martin is a physician who counsels many other people about their recovery. As a stroke survivor, he now has the opportunity to reflect on his own recovery. He agrees with Alice that the key is to "do things that you can be successful at, concentrate on your assets, not on your deficits. Do things you think you have power to do." Martin suggested that loss of control is loss of power: "We need to work on having the power back. We lost power and control and self-esteem [when we had our strokes]. Anything that anyone can do to help us get these back is helpful." In essence, he suggested that the connection Alice made between a sense of self-worth, on the one hand, and persistent and patient accomplishment of small achievements, on the other hand, is central to a successful recovery process. He finds this lesson to be validated not only through the work he has done with his patients, but also through his own hard-fought recovery.

The National Stroke Association (1986) seems to make the same assumptions as Alice and Martin regarding the importance of a sense of self-worth and persistence. This association suggests that developing a plan of action and a specific set of tangible goals "can help restore the capacity to make decisions and execute choices" (p. 43). Developing a plan and establishing goals can also encourage the stroke survivor's return to old hobbies and interests as well as the identification of new interests, strengths, and abilities. The National Stroke Association recommends that the stroke survivor and family set four types of goals. First, *physical rehabilitation* goals should be established that incorporate plans for exercise, weight loss (if appropriate), and diet. This plan should be built in conjunction with the medical and rehabilitation teams. Second, *social and recreational* goals should be identified and plans made for the survivor to participate in enjoyable and supportive activities—usually including a local stroke club or support group. We would suggest that similar plans be established for the primary caregiver. This person also needs support and must not become isolated. Third, the National Stroke Association recommends *family and community* goals. These allow each family member, close friend, and local community agency to contribute to the recovery process. Focusing on family and community goals not only maximizes the support the survivor receives but also often helps to restore or improve family relationships, friendships, and even ties with community groups (such as the estranged relationship between John and his church congregation). Fourth, a set of *personal* goals should be established that move the survivor toward greater independence and a greater sense of self-worth. These personal goals may range from learning to tie one's shoelaces again, to resumption of driving, to taking on a new hobby or community activity.

Sheila would undoubtedly agree with Alice, Martin, and the National Stroke Association on the importance of these goals. Sheila believes that one must be patient and celebrate the little victories as a stroke survivor. She stated that her stroke taught her to take a no-nonsense approach to life. She learned that it takes time to work on things every day. Don't give up. She would say to those who have lost their ability to speak, "So you can never talk . . . use pictures to communicate. There are always other ways to do things." Sheila would let other stroke survivors know that they can relearn the things they did before their stroke. However, it takes longer and sometimes they will get it right, but not always. She would then ask them, "What else do you have to do?" Keep moving along. Don't give up. Try the little things. Perfect them but recognize that you will never be able to do them right every time. There will always be some failures; however, the only ultimate failure is not trying!

The Right Balance Between Challenge and Support

The lessons that many of our stroke survivors—in particular, our fe-male survivors—have taught us about the value of self-respect and per-severance must be balanced against the equally great need for support and assistance. Jane does a superb job of balancing challenge and sup-port. She continues to challenge herself by returning to work and by actively exercising. "Going back to work was very important," she noted. Also, "if I don't exercise, my body feels funny . . . I feel like exercise is the most important part . . . walking, getting out of the house. . . . Have people take you out, get out of the house, even just to a show." She couples these challenging activities with a strong dose of support, through attending a stroke club. Jane claimed that being with other survivors helps her confront her fear and frustration. In the stroke group, she not only receives support from others but also is able to offer sup-port and understanding to them, which is affirming for her.

Beth, too, repeatedly spoke of the need for balance between chal-lenge and support. With regard to appropriate support, she pointed to the importance of receiving adequate psychological services at the hospi-tal and later at home. She received no assistance from the hospital other than medical treatment and suggested that hospitals should have a pam-phlet describing all the services in the community that are available for stroke survivors. This pamphlet should include fees, whether or not Medicare provides reimbursement, and how to get to the services by public transportation. Beth did not find out about her local stroke club for approximately a year. When she attended her initial meeting, it was the first time she'd said, "I had a stroke." She avails herself of other support services as well: an exercise class for stroke survivors, senior citizens' activities, and an informal morning walking group.

Beth also frequently mentioned with appreciation the support her family offered. Nevertheless, she described several incidents when they wanted to do too much for her. In these cases, she wanted a little less support and a little more challenge. An example was her desire to take the bus to her doctor's appointment at the hospital, so that she could spend time in the gift shop and do some window shopping afterward.

Her children wanted to drive her to the appointment, but she explained that she had never driven and thought it was important to continue to ride the bus. In this way, she maintained something from her life prior to the stroke while also asserting her poststroke independence.

Support from Other People

Ironically, while many of the women we interviewed concluded that the stroke experience forced or encouraged them to become more self-assertive and independent, the men typically learned the often-hard lesson of relying more on the support and assistance of others. The women frequently had been in a dependent role or had spent years caring for others. Now, at the point when they are most vulnerable, they most want (and need) to assert their independence and develop a sense of self-worth. The men, by contrast, have often spent their lives asserting their independence. They have worked hard to be autonomous but now in midlife are faced with stroke-induced disabilities that force them back into dependency. Often the stressful life-style they embraced in an effort to become more independent has led them to this new dependency. Important lessons are to be learned from both the men and women we interviewed.

Like Alice and Sheila, Sean acknowledged that the major lesson he learned concerns his own sense of self-worth and perseverance. However, unlike Alice and Sheila, he also pointed to the importance of friends and professional counselors. Sean now goes to two stroke clubs, has close male friends in whom he confides, and has begun group psychotherapy. Prior to joining the psychotherapy group, Sean saw a psychiatrist for several months. He is also in two support groups that relate to his job search (both of which he had started before his stroke).

Sean seems to approach his emotional recovery from the stroke with the same thoroughness that produced his rapid physical recovery—an achievement he contrasted with one doctor's prognosis that "full recovery may take years." Sean did not want to believe the doctor's words. With the recovery of some physical functions, he was able to regain self-esteem and become more patient about his continuing recovery. Sean acknowledged the damaging effects of his prestroke perfectionism, self-reliance, and driven life-style. He believes that the stroke forced him to question and ultimately abandon this life-style in favor of a more connected, supportive way of life. This illustrates, yet again, the unanticipated insights and benefits gained from the successful adaptation to a stroke.

Like Sean, Todd recommended that other stroke survivors "get a support group and be around people who understand what you are going through." According to Todd, his closest friends are like him in that they are workaholics. Furthermore, like Todd, they tend to deny that they are driven and highly stressed. He continues to be frustrated about their failure to heed his warnings about slowing down and taking care of themselves. Todd offers himself as an example but hears their denial when he reminds them of their mortality. He recognizes his own defensiveness in other people around him, and like John and many other stroke survivors, appreciates the message that his stroke delivered in a forcible manner to him: slow down or die!

Another male survivor—Tom—similarly acknowledged (indirectly) the important lessons he learned about the value of support offered by other people. When his interviewer asked him about what he would like to tell other stroke survivors, Tom stated, "Damned if I know. I can't figure it out for myself." After the interview, Tom and the interviewer chatted casually for a few minutes. The interviewer then thanked him and stood up to leave. Tom stopped the interviewer and said, "I'm really glad you came and I hope you'll come back. No one stops anymore, and no one has ever asked me how I felt about my stroke."

This concluding remark certainly contains an important lesson. Why hasn't anyone ever talked with him about his stroke? Did they think that it would be too painful for him? Tom has made it clear that he would rather talk through the pain than remain isolated. Perhaps no one talks with him because they feel powerless to help him through this process—or because if they were to talk about the stroke, it would remind them of how vulnerable they are, too. Yet Tom has suggested that simply listening to him can be healing. Listening is an expression of concern and commitment. Furthermore, he gets to talk about something important to him. He gets to test out his reality and determine if he is "insane" or perhaps just a little frightened. An alternative reason for Tom's isolation may be that no one cares enough to spend time with him. If so, Tom has taught us all a poignant lesson: some stroke survivors are deserted physically or at least emotionally by their family and friends and need someone else to talk to. Tom's dilemma points to the important role played by various support groups, community volunteer programs, and other human service activities directed toward isolated stroke survivors.

PART FOUR

Helping the Survivor

12

Family Caregivers
Tell Their Stories

The experiences at the time of the stroke are certainly frightening
and disorienting for the person suffering from the stroke. Physical
pain, cortical misfirings, paralysis, blindness, and hearing loss all contribute to the pervasive and awesome experience of everything going
wrong at the same time. The people who are most intimately affiliated
with the person having the stroke also experience the stroke as shocking, frightening, and often beyond their understanding about the nature of "typical" medical problems. Everything seems to be going wrong
with someone they care about deeply. What could be more disconcerting?

In this chapter, we focus specifically on the caregivers' experience
of the stroke, looking as we did in previous chapters not only at the
stroke experience itself but also at the slow and often frustrating (and
sometimes rewarding) processes of rehabilitation and recovery. We turn
first to the caregivers' experiences of the stroke itself.

The Nightmare Begins

Tina was fifty-four years old when Parker had his stroke. They had been
married for thirty-two years (virtually all their adult lives). She was with
Parker in the morning when his vision became blurred and went with
him to the doctor to see what was wrong. They were told that everything looked fine, and he went home—only to have a stroke. Later that
day, she saw the same doctor at the hospital where Parker was taken

after he suffered the stroke. She recalls screaming at this doctor, blaming him for the stroke and threatening him physically. She has since apologized to the physician—but in this moment of anger, Tina expressed the feelings experienced by many stroke survivors: she was angry, felt betrayed, and didn't know what was happening to Parker or to herself. Someone should have known what was going to happen! Someone should have warned her or Parker! Someone is responsible for this horrible thing that just happened to a person I love and have lived with most of my life!

The experience for Mary, the caregiver, and Ralph, her husband, was different in some ways; yet in other ways she too felt confused, angry, and perhaps betrayed. When Ralph had his stroke, he had no pain because he passed out and fell. Mary was at home and phoned for help. She knew the signs of a stroke and immediately recognized his symptoms. When he became conscious, Mary said she could hardly tell he had had a stroke. He awoke before the ambulance arrived, and they had difficulty convincing him to go to the hospital. Only one person on the ambulance team was knowledgeable about strokes. Therefore, Ralph and Mary decided to go to the hospital in a truck. Before arriving at the hospital, he suffered another stroke. In retrospect, both Ralph and Mary wish he had taken the ambulance.

Ralph's prognosis was poor from the start. The hospital personnel performed three brain scans. The stroke was not apparent until the third scan. Ralph spent two days in telemetry (the hospital unit where heart patients are monitored continuously), had no control over either his legs or left arm, and had difficulty articulating words. On the third day after the stroke, Mary was discouraged when a physician at the hospital said, "He's not going to be much better than this for the rest of his life." Their own physician gave them the most useful information about the stroke. Mary spoke of the benefits of having a regular physician work with a stroke survivor. During this crisis, it was helpful to have the communication and trust already established with a physician.

Bea was also physically present when Ted had his stroke. However, unlike Mary, Bea was afraid, having known little at the time about strokes or about the recovery process. She was able to cope with her fear, however, by taking life a day at a time. She found herself apprehensive at times—looking for any signs of another stroke. Taking Ted to the hospital and not knowing what was going on was traumatic for Bea. She was in shock when she looked at how her life had changed in one crashing moment and at what she would be dealing with in the future. At the time, she later reported, she was feeling the need to remain calm despite the situation.

The feelings of fear and even terror are not confined to Bea or the other female caregivers we interviewed. For Benjamin, the experience of Dorothy's stroke was frightening. He remembers her not being able to move or talk and described it as a bleak moment in his life. Ben really felt he was going to lose her. After Dorothy had been in the hospital for eight days, a neurosurgeon told Benjamin that she had a strong possibility for a 90 percent recovery and that he should place her in a rehabilitation center (rather than a convalescent center) so that the goal would be recovery. He was relieved and began planning the recovery process. This was not easy because other relatives intervened and placed her in a convalescent hospital instead. Ben and Dorothy had only been married for three years when she had her stroke. As a result, he was not able to gain the support or understanding of Dorothy's family. He persevered, however, and Dorothy was eventually placed in a rehabilitation center. This story of both despair and hope speaks to the value of professional medical advice—especially when it is based on the welfare of the stroke survivor and a sense that poststroke rehabilitation is the given, rather than traditional convalescence.

Since people who have strokes tend to be older, our interviewees were often retired and more sedentary, hence were home with their caregiver when the stroke occurred. In a few instances, however, the stroke occurred when the caregiver was not present. Patricia, for example, has been married to Otto for sixty-three years and they spend most of their time together. Yet she was not physically present when Otto had his stroke. She was out shopping and returned home to find him standing up but holding onto the back of a chair. She asked him what was wrong and he said, "I think I had a stroke." He put his hand to his head and indicated that it had felt like something had hit him in the head. He then collapsed, and Patricia went to the phone, calling her son to come over to help her take Otto to the hospital.

Knowledge that a stroke has occurred is invaluable. Otto's recognition of the symptoms of strokes undoubtedly was useful to Patricia in deciding on a course of action. This knowledge, however, does not eliminate or even reduce the powerful emotional states (fear, confusion, anger) that caregivers typically experience when a loved one has suffered a stroke. Even if they know that a stroke has occurred, they know little about its severity or about the probable impact of this event on their own life or the life of their loved one. Knowledge, in other words, is no substitute for emotional support. Both are needed if caregivers are to be effective in the role they have suddenly assumed in the life of this significant other person.

Patricia felt helpless in part because she knew that she couldn't lift Otto by herself, so she had to wait until her son arrived. Otto did regain consciousness, so Patricia and her son were able to assist him to the car and take him to the hospital. Patricia stated during her interview that she was relieved when her son arrived. However, when they got to the hospital, no one spoke to her about Otto's condition, except to tell her that he had had a stroke. Unfortunately, this is more information than many caregivers receive. Three days passed before anyone told her the extent of Otto's medical problems. She was given a list of available community resources, but she does not remember anyone talking to her about the psychological implications of the stroke or the physical demands it would make of her. She emphasized that there would have been no way anyone could have prepared her for these dramatic changes in her life. She thought something like this could never happen.

Once again, knowledge is not sufficient. It can never adequately prepare one for the shifts in life that will occur. There must be personal support during the transitional period, though information is still a necessary condition to make the support possible. Without adequate information, a caregiver will be that much more anxious and confused; emotional support will serve primarily as an inadequate Band-Aid rather than as a valuable resource. The coupling of information and support is essential if caregiving is to be successful.

Caregiving is frequently provided by someone close to the stroke survivor other than a spouse. In the case of our interviewees, the caregiver was often a daughter, daughter-in-law, or son of the survivor. Dan is the fifty-four-year-old son of a seventy-nine-year-old woman, Anna, who has experienced many other tragic events in her life in addition to having had a stroke. Her oldest son and grandson were killed in an automobile accident, and several years later, her husband was shot and killed during an armed robbery of his gas station. Shortly thereafter, she experienced the first of three strokes. And her youngest son recently died at forty-two years of age of a massive heart attack.

Dan is a divorced father of three teenage sons and lives approximately three hours from his mother. They talk on the telephone every day, and he spends his two days off each week with her. At this time, he cleans house, takes her to the doctor, does her banking, and generally assists her with her daily living activities. Recently, he has arranged for someone to do domestic work several hours each day. He is very concerned since his mother is alone at night and for periods of time each day. He did live further away when his mother had her first stroke. They had no warning of the first stroke, and Dan is thankful that a female cousin was able to provide substantial assistance until he could move closer to his mother.

For Dan, the experience of living through his mother's strokes was particularly painful and disturbing: "It brought back painful memories of my father's and brothers' deaths. I thought she would die immediately. I adjusted when I saw that she was still alive. It would have been hard to lose my mother. I prayed she would not succumb to death." Dan also stated that "the guilt would have been hard to overcome— not seeing my mother for more than two to three times per year after being around them all the time when I was growing up."

Like many caregivers (and particularly those who are not the spouse of the stroke survivor), Dan said he was told little about his mother's condition when he arrived at the hospital. The doctor did mention that she had a stroke, that the next forty-eight hours would tell more, and that he would just have to wait. After two days, they informed him she was out of danger and indicated that she would need an operation.

However, no further details or explanations were provided. The physician might have told Dan what he could expect in terms of recovery and how he might be of help. Information regarding other resources available to assist in the rehabilitation process would also have been valuable in reassuring Dan and supplementing his own efforts.

Kevin and Leonard are a gay couple who have been together for twenty years. Kevin is sixty-seven and had his stroke two years before the interview was conducted. He was at the breakfast table and just slumped to the floor. As in the case of Mary, Leonard was familiar with the signs of a stroke: "I knew it was a stroke immediately. Naturally, I was concerned and afraid. It was the worst day of my life." As with Mary, knowledge about strokes helps but does not ease the pain associated with the unknown outcomes: "You feel fear—rather, terror in my case. You don't know what to do or what is going to happen. You're almost helpless. Then you just do what you need to do. . . . It was six or seven hours before we got a room in the hospital. Kevin was on a gurney in the emergency room and the hallway during that entire time. I was furious at [the hospital staff]. I was [also] afraid because . . . the doctors . . . either talked as if Kevin was a plant or wasn't there at all."

The problems associated with fear of the unknown were intensified in many instances by a lack of sufficient information from the hospital staff. As we have noted throughout this book, many stroke survivors and caregivers feel that they did not receive adequate information or received it before they were able to process it. It is perhaps understandable that medical staff are reluctant to speak with stroke survivors immediately after their arrival at the hospital, given their confused state of mind. But what about the caregivers? They are anxious and confused, but some of this can be reduced with a little information. Unfortunately, caregivers all too often indicated during their interview that they learned little of value from the hospital staff. Sylvia said that she was told nothing about the nature and prognosis of her husband's physical condition until several days after his stroke. She specifically asked Steven's physician for some information about strokes but was told only the bare minimum—that her husband had had a stroke. The hospital staff were not much more helpful during his two months of hospitalization. She finally managed to get detailed information from an outpatient rehabilitation facility.

Betty also received frustratingly little information after John's stroke. She emphasizes that she, as a caregiver, should have been told (1) what to expect by way of "normal" or average progress, (2) how to handle the emotional reactions (on her part and her husband's), (3) the nature of the rehabilitation process—particularly its slow pace and the need for patience, and (4) the importance of looking beyond the discharge from physical therapy when identifying treatment goals. We would add three other items that should be provided, based on the suggestions of other caregivers: (5) a list of resources available in the local community for both stroke survivors and caregivers, (6) material stressing the importance of family, friends, and other groups (for example, church, social club, work) in providing logistical and emotional support, and (7) information on the appropriateness and location of professional counseling for both survivors and caregivers.

Being of Help

Mary was constantly in attendance at both the hospital and the convalescent home while Ralph was recovering from his stroke. She said it was necessary to be there to advocate for him. After two months, he was released from the convalescent hospital. Mary described his release as premature and felt that the hospital staff had abandoned them. She prepared as well as she could for Ralph's return, replacing the carpet with one with a low nap and replacing their mattress with a new firm one. Friends rallied to build ramps for the house.

Mary feels that caregivers are usually not prepared for the challenges when a stroke survivor returns home. On arriving home from the convalescent hospital, Mary got Ralph out of the car and proceeded to shuttle him up the driveway by placing a chair several yards away and having him alternate a few steps with sitting and resting. She would move the chair as he stood to walk. After getting him to the house, she thought, "I don't know if I can handle this." In the two years following the stroke, the tension in the back of Mary's neck has spread to both arms. At times, this has been paralyzing. She also experiences extreme fatigue. Her sleep is regularly disturbed, because she needs to change the bed once or twice per night. In spite of these obstacles, she seems strong and determined—a woman with definite goals. During the interview, her strengths were readily apparent and yet she did not acknowledge them. She stated that "I have to do it. I am going to do it." Her goal is for Ralph to become self-sufficient. He spoke lovingly and with admiration of his wife's support and patience. She, conversely, described herself as impatient and mean to Ralph when tired.

Like Mary, Sylvia is a strong, persistent caregiver. She attributes much of this strength to her religious faith. As soon as her husband, Steven, had his stroke, Sylvia called her church: "It was difficult, but I prayed and left everything up to God." Knowing how Steven had lived his life as a very active and successful businessperson, Sylvia prayed that he would be able to cope with whatever kind of life was left for him: "I accepted everything as it came day to day and tried to go from there." She added, "I really think that Steven took it as well as he did because of those sincere prayers from the church group." Regardless of what one thinks of the effectiveness of prayer, it is clear that the church group was a wonderful source of immediate support for both Steven and Sylvia. It is often the caregiver who is most in need of this broad-based community support, since the stroke survivor usually receives the undivided attention of the caregiver.

Tina only gradually opened up regarding the challenges associated with taking care of her husband during the recovery period. She eventually talked, with some relief, about frustrations with family and friends, with the recovery process, and with her husband, Parker. While her family and friends claim she has turned into a "grumpy old lady" who doesn't do anything, those same people don't offer to sit with Parker for lengthy periods of time nor do they invite the two of them out. Tina resents the fact that their friends have "abandoned" them and that their children don't really understand what it takes to care for their father day in and day out. Financially, they could afford a visiting nurse, but Parker hates the idea and has gotten very depressed when Tina leaves him.

Tina claims to have accepted the stroke. She doubts Parker will get much better, but she doesn't want him to lose hope. Acceptance was very hard, because they had fought and overcome an earlier auto accident (Parker crashed during an auto race and burned 80 percent of his body). They initially both thought Parker's stroke was going to be defeated, just as he had recovered, with Tina's help, from the accident: "After the burns, [Parker's] recovery was so miraculous and this has been so disappointing." For Tina, the accident produced a few positive changes in their lives. Parker was more settled and more committed to their marriage and to his children; since the stroke, however, Tina feels that she must constantly push Parker, using sarcasm or ignoring him when he won't even try to complete the simplest task by himself: "I have become a grumpy old lady [as her family accuses her of being] and I don't like it."

Tina is frustrated, but she knows it isn't anyone's fault. She holds little hope that someday she will look back and see any positive outcomes from the stroke. She has slowly and painfully realized that while Parker eventually recovered from the burns, he is never going to completely recover from the stroke. She knows that many of the aftereffects of a stroke are permanent and has resigned herself to playing the role of caregiver for the rest of Parker's life. Such a recognition is inevitably painful and stressful. Tina (and Parker) must grieve for a life that will never return and directly face the new challenges of limited recovery and caregiving.

Initially, Tina and Parker were given a time frame for recovery by their attending physician. Tina believes now that this was the wrong thing to do: "People set their hopes on those times and when you don't recover it is so sad." Yet other caregivers speak about the value of information and receiving realistic expectations regarding probable degree of recovery and length of time for rehabilitation. What is the right amount of information to receive from medical authorities and when is the best time for the caregiver (and stroke survivor) to receive this information?

Like many other caregivers, Patricia wished that she had received more information about how to prepare for her caregiving role and more assistance during the early stages of her husband's rehabilitation, given the problems she has experienced with her husband, Otto, during this period. She got very frustrated and angry with Otto's unwillingness to allow nurses or other outside caretakers to come in and help her. Patricia feels he used his physical condition as an excuse to withdraw and avoid doing things for himself. She indicated that the mornings used to be (and in many instances still are) the worst time for her, because Otto needs constant custodial care. She says she feels like a "nag" having to push and remind him to get up and come to breakfast. She worries about being too harsh with him, especially when she feels tired or over-whelmed. Like virtually all of the other caregivers, she feels that the situation is extremely demanding, both physically and emotionally. She says that at times she really resents his total dependence on her.

During Ted's recovery period, Bea had to make a number of changes in her own life. She considers the most important change to be one of managing their finances. Bea used to leave the finances up to Ted. Now she must manage the money, as well as helping Ted with many other decisions, thereby (at least in her own mind) "robbing him" of what he did for a long period of time. Ted now does things around the house that Bea used to do, such as setting the table in the morning and helping to get breakfast. That makes him feel useful. Neverthe-less, these are not traditional "male" roles, and they leave him feeling incompetent.

As noted earlier, we found that family members other than spouses frequently serve as caregivers. Often this caregiving by another family member is fraught with resistance or resentment—typically directed toward relatives who are not doing their fair share of the caregiving or are trying to move the treatment program in a different direction. Ellen is the daughter-in-law of Teresa, yet she provides much more of the care for Teresa than do any of Teresa's three children or other family members. Teresa doesn't protest that Ellen is providing most of the care, for she knows that she needs help from her family and that her chil-dren have put Ellen in charge. Furthermore, Teresa senses that it is in her best interest to please Ellen and to cooperate, even if this means denial of her personal feelings. Ellen also does a lot of denying about her own emotions regarding Teresa. When the interviewer brought up Teresa's incontinence, Ellen quickly noted that this is "the least of our worries now."

Ellen is aware of Teresa's underlying resistance to her well-meant caregiving. In spite of the power vested in her by other family members, Ellen says that she feels powerless and frustrated at times: "I can't control what Teresa does. She listens to her daughter Sally, who constantly pulls her mother in the opposite direction by telling her she doesn't have to do this or that." *Control* is an important word in Ellen's vocabulary. She sees herself as having been in a managing role since she was fifteen, when her mother died and she took over the household, including the care of three younger siblings. She married Teresa's son, Arnie, at age eighteen. Now the mother of two children, she also works as a bookkeeper: "I've always been active and organized."

It did not surprise Ellen that the family turned to her when Teresa had her stroke. She proudly described herself as "the family planner, organizer, and mediator." She indicated that "somebody had to take charge of the situation." She was the one who kept her cool when the others reacted with confusion and indecision. It was Ellen who convinced Teresa that she needed to go to the hospital (it took her two hours to break through Teresa's denial). It was Ellen who called the doctor, insisted on immediate action, demanded that certain tests be done, and arranged for hospitalization as well as placement in a rehabilitation facility and follow-up care at home. The family also left it to Ellen to deal with the insurance company and negotiate with doctors and nurses.

In contrast to the immobilizing shock experienced by other family members, Ellen's reaction was "relief" when Teresa had her last stroke—the latest of three attacks. This was the proof she needed to convince the doctor that something was wrong with Teresa and that something needed to be done. She bristles with anger as she recalls the lack of attention Teresa got from the doctor after Teresa's first two strokes: "There were signs and symptoms that were ignored by the doctor. That was just not acceptable to me."

Ellen recalls her role in the drama with a mixture of triumph and anger. Her vehement reaction to her mother-in-law's stroke is out of sync with her detachment. There is no display of tenderness toward Teresa, no outward sign of caring, except in the efficiency with which she manages Teresa's care. She has typed up a list that spells out Teresa's daily activities almost to the minute. She is knowledgeable about Teresa's medications, exercises, and diet. She had an electronic alarm system installed in the house to assure Teresa of immediate help in case of another stroke. But there does not seem to be the kind of emotional attachment between them that we found between many of the other stroke survivors and caregivers we interviewed or that would seem to justify Ellen's passionate response to Teresa's stroke. Ellen's emotional reaction seems more understandable when seen in connection with her helplessness in the face of her own mother's illness and death.

At the present time, Teresa's family does not seem to be adequately equipped emotionally to deal with her stroke recovery. They have left virtually all of the caregiving to a daughter-in-law who is emotionally detached from Teresa and seems to be working out issues from her own adolescence rather than dealing directly with her relationship with Teresa or other members of Teresa's immediate family. Unless the family comes to grips with the need for shared responsibility regarding Teresa's recovery, Ellen's energetic determination is likely to continue to fill in for genuine emotional commitment. Other members of the family will remain passive and probably feel thankful, guilty, and resentful of Ellen's controlling manner. Teresa will continue to feel helpless and probably resentful (at an unexpressed level) of Ellen's controlling, dispassionate attention. She will continue to do as she is told by Ellen and will find little motivation to become more independent and self-confident. Teresa has grown depressed and is not responding well to treatment. Hopefully, she will find a stroke support group in which she can have permission to work through her losses and resentment about lack of genuine family support.

In Dan's case—as the son of a stroke survivor—there were no options regarding caregiving, for his father and two other siblings had died before his mother, Anna, had her first stroke. The major problem for Dan was the resentment of his sons to the time demands his mother was making on him. Everywhere Dan turned, he faced familial demands and an attendant sense of guilt. As the primary caregiver for his mother, he felt he helped as much as he could—living three hours from her. He indicated that he is sorry that she has to live out her golden years as a bitter and financially impoverished person. He claimed that his mother has locked herself up in the house and will not come out. That has had a definite ripple effect in Dan's life, since he has had to spend all of his spare time taking care of her while neglecting his teenage sons who live near him.

Dan has somehow coped with the situation by trying to keep realistic expectations about how much he can do: "I've never felt I was Florence Nightingale." The most important thing he has accomplished as a caregiver was arranging for someone to take care of his mother and her household chores. He realized that he could not be with his mother all the time and knew that someone had to be there to watch over her. He does feel that it is a son's responsibility to take care of his mother— "especially if he is the last son."

Throughout the interview, recurring themes of guilt were expressed. He feels guilty if he is not at his mother's home more often than he was before her stroke. This was particularly stressful when he thought that she might soon die. He sees his relationship with his mother and with his sons as those of sacrifice: a sacrifice of the young to the old, or of the old to the young. Who gets short shrift, his aging and disabled mother or his dependent and needy sons? Dan seems to have made the decision that he can lose a few months with his sons without a lasting effect. His mother, however, requires and warrants his time and care during this period in her life: "There are times when you do what you have to do and hope people will be understanding."

Dan feels he can now be with and talk to his mother and not run away as he did when he was younger: "I handle the cleaning chores, gardening, run errands, buy groceries, and feel happy about it. I do what she gave me as a child. I am now able to give back to her as an adult." Much as many women feel that their husbands become like children when recovering from a stroke, Dan sees that his mother has become like a child and he like a parent. In this way, he can "return the favor" of his own childhood and perhaps ameliorate some of the guilt associated with early adulthood neglect of his mother (as well as, perhaps, the guilt associated with relative neglect of his now-deceased father and brothers during this period in his life).

Meeting the Needs of Caregivers

Given these diverse and often-disturbing accounts of caregiving, what do these men and women seem to need? First, caregivers require some caregiving themselves. While a spouse or child might assume primary responsibility for taking care of a stroke survivor, other members of the family, friends, and those in the human service professions must, in turn, provide the caregivers with timely information, practical assistance, and emotional support. The stories we heard suggest that all too often, caregivers are lost in the rehabilitation process. Everyone focuses on the survivors and ignores the people who must be there everyday for them. In Rod McLean's case, we should ask, Who was providing support for his parents and fiancée, given that they were always there to support his efforts? We can't expect the stroke survivors to provide this support, since they are in the midst of struggling with their own issues. Other people must be there as part of an extended support network.

Second, caregivers need a safe place in which to talk about their own experiences. They often feel uncomfortable talking about their frustrations and fears sitting next to the person they are caring for in a stroke group. They need their own support group, comprised of other people like themselves who have been suddenly thrust into the difficult role of caring for someone to whom they are deeply attached. Human service agencies that provide stroke group services should schedule some separate meetings for the caregivers and should encourage them to attend these meetings. Because many feel guilty about leaving their partners alone or with someone else, the caregiver support groups should be scheduled in conjunction with special activities for the stroke survivors.

Third, most caregivers are also in need of more mundane assistance: housekeeping, occasional cooking, and often some nursing. They often have to do the work around their house that they once shared with their spouse or, at the very least, they now have less time than before to do chores they have done for many years. Once again, family members and friends can be of great help, either in providing these services themselves or in contributing some money so that the caregiver can hire someone to help out around the house or in nursing the stroke survivor. Even if the latter course is taken, it is still critical that family members and friends help to "spell" a caregiver on occasion, so that they can do their own chores or simply get out of the house to enjoy themselves, while the stroke survivor is being looked after by someone they know and trust.

Finally, it is also clear from the interviews that a stroke often has a profound impact not only on the stroke survivor and caregiver but also on their relationship—particularly when the stroke survivor is relying exclusively on the caregiver for support and care. Long-married couples often find that their relationship must change, which requires readjusting old, established, and often quite gratifying roles, responsibilities, and habitual ways of interacting with one another. In some cases, the relationship is sufficiently flexible and sturdy so that the partners can negotiate the changes themselves. In other cases, the relationship isn't sturdy or is highly inflexible. In yet other cases, the survivor or the caregiver or both have created such a dependent relationship that the caregiver assumes total responsibility for the rehabilitation process, often isolating the survivor and making this person less motivated to assume responsibility for his or her own recovery.

If the relationship isn't strong, if it already is burdened by major problems, if the caregiver is exclusively responsible for the rehabilitation, or if the rehabilitation is particularly stressful, the recovery process and the health of the relationship are likely to be in jeopardy and negatively impacted by each other. In these instances, couples may need some marital counseling or therapy or (in the case of parent-child caregiving) family counseling or therapy. If the relationship doesn't weather the impact of the stroke, both the stroke survivor and the caregiver are likely to find the process of recovery difficult if not impossible.

13

—

Learning from
Family Caregivers

E very caregiver we interviewed talked about the dramatic changes
in their lives as the result of their loved one's stroke and the new
role they assumed as caregiver. In virtually all cases, major losses were
associated with the stroke and the caregiving role—a loss of freedom,
of companionship, of future dreams regarding such diverse activities
as traveling, participating in the arts, initiating joint projects, or engaging in active grandparenting. In many instances, it was surprising
to discover some gains from the stroke as well. The stroke survivor became emotionally more accessible, the caregiver was able to assume
more control or responsibility in the home, or the stroke survivor and
caregiver drew closer together in their joint efforts at rehabilitation.

At the heart of the matter was the opportunity of the caregiver
to explore new avenues of development and new ways of relating to
the survivor. Caregiving responsibilities are never something we ask
for, but when we are confronted with the need to care for another person, we can choose to define this as an opportunity for personal growth
and new learning. Shimberg (1990, p. 204) concludes her book on
caregiving with just such a sentiment: "There is life and love after a
stroke. There also is a great deal of learning, as much for the family
as for the stroke survivor. We measure days to their fullest now, seeking joy and contentment in our today rather than waiting for any tomor-
rows. And we keep turning corners to prevent looking back to what
was." Each of the caregivers we interviewed told a different story, though

there were repeated themes of both gain and loss and similarities in lessons learned. We turn in this chapter to these issues and to the personal, often emotionally charged experiences of caregivers as they confronted their own needs, hopes, and fears in their new poststroke reality.

Gains and Losses for Caregivers

For Karen, the times just before her husband, Derrin, had his stroke were some of the best in their marriage. Derrin had just retired, their finances were in good shape, and they did a lot of traveling. Karen was still working full time. Thus, the stroke was devastating for her, and she experienced many losses as a result of this traumatic event. There were no warning signs, which made their life changes more abrupt and difficult to handle. Like many other caregivers, Karen spoke of being married to a "new person" after the stroke. She even went so far as to identify two marriages—one that lasted for forty-one years and a second marriage (to the same man) that has so far lasted four years.

Fortunately, Karen has received considerable assistance from her family, which has enabled her at least not to lose her career. She has been able to keep busy in her job, which has made the adjustments in her marriage a bit more bearable. At first, the changes were particularly difficult. Her family didn't know what to do. Derrin's physicians offered neither information nor support. Karen spent almost all of her free time with Derrin and resented the hospital staff's suggestions that she was spending too much time at the hospital, that he didn't need her constant attention, and that she should take better care of herself. She felt at that time that she knew what Derrin really wanted. He wanted them to be together all the time.

In some ways, Karen's relationship with Derrin hasn't changed much since he was in the hospital. In other ways, there have been major changes—for the better. They still spend a lot of time together. During the interview, she sat just outside the room in view of Derrin and the interviewer, listening to what he said and occasionally interjecting comments. This tended to restrict Derrin's ability to respond freely to the questions being asked. At the beginning of the interview, Karen had gone outside for a while and Derrin seemed to speak much more freely. What is it like for Derrin to always have Karen around monitoring his behavior? On the one hand, he must be pleased that she cares so much about him. On the other hand, is he receiving too much support and not enough challenge? Perhaps the hospital staff was right in suggesting that Karen was spending too much time with him.

Karen indicated that during the first year after the stroke, Derrin was very abusive toward her. He was angry that she had taken over so many things that he could do before and that she could still move about with ease. She says that now he is a nicer person than he was immediately after the stroke. Perhaps this is because Karen no longer attempts to do everything for him, though obviously she is still monitoring his conversations (at least with the interviewer). She eventually realized that she had to walk out of the room when he dressed himself, so that she would not try to help him out. In this way, he learned to dress himself. He has recovered at least some of the functions and responsibilities he carried out prior to the stroke.

Karen's role in the family has definitely changed since the stroke, even though Derrin has assumed some of his former duties. She used to be just "mom" to her children. Now she is the person they come to for decision making; however, they don't ask for her advice in front of their father. She sees herself as stronger, sharper, and "nastier" in getting things done. She misses being able to share problems, dance, and walk together with Derrin. His mind is "a little muddled" so she can't solve problems with Derrin, although she did try that at first. He would say, "You deal with it." She misses having time for herself as well as the independence she formerly took for granted.

Tina similarly spoke of the loss of free time as a result of Parker's stroke. His stroke has left her without any private or free time. She feels that she can relax only when Parker is asleep—and she admits to resenting this: "It's like when you are raising children. Only after you put them to bed do you get a moment's peace." Their days are filled with a constant round of medical appointments for the stroke, for the hip, for diabetes. They go to physical therapy and group therapy. This schedule takes an emotional and physical toll on both of them.

Prior to the stroke, Parker was semiretired and they went camping and fishing regularly. Now, he doesn't even want to go for a drive in the mountains. As was the case with most of the other couples we interviewed, Parker had been very dominating prior to his stroke and Tina had accepted this conservative male role. She has found her shift to the more "masculine" role of financial manager difficult: "I don't like challenge. I was very content." The current nature of their relationship, as with many couples, resembles a hovering parent and dependent child. They are both aware of these changes, and neither Parker nor Tina likes it. Neither, however, can foresee their circumstances improving so that they could get back to their old, more comfortable roles. Unlike many of the other female caregivers we interviewed, Tina does not believe that these new responsibilities have made her stronger, nor does she think she has grown as a person in general because of the stroke. Tina has begrudgingly constructed a new self—though she has little time to do anything other than attend to her husband's needs.

For Tina and Parker, the stroke recovery process and the caregiving role have become problematic in large part because of their inability to move out of traditional marital roles. Men are supposed to be taken care of, and women are supposed to be the caregivers. In her study of the relationship between race, culture, and stroke recovery, Zelman (1992) points out that these problems are particularly common and exacerbated in traditional cultures. In many Asian American, black, and Hispanic communities, "There is a moral imperative to care for stroke survivors at home within the family" (Zelman, 1992, p. 4). Economic necessities often compound the problem. These families simply can't afford outside help—as is also the case with many other families, regardless of race or culture. While this moral imperative is no longer as pronounced as it used to be, a strong tendency to avoid outside assistance survives in these communities, and the spouse (particularly the wife) is often still expected to take primary responsibility for all caregiving. Fortunately, these communities also encourage broad-based participation among other family members in the caregiving function, thus reducing the chances that the primary caregiver will become overburdened and isolated.

In contrast to the experience of Tina and Parker and many other couples we interviewed, the period of recovery for Benjamin and Dorothy tended to strengthen rather than weaken their relationship. Perhaps the outcomes were more positive because Ben and Dorothy had been married for only three years at the time of Dorothy's stroke. Dorothy says that Ben is her hero. She wakes up at night and is so grateful that he is there to help her. She says that he does things you would not expect a husband of his generation to do. Ben has been through an unusually difficult year—not only with Dorothy's stroke and the loss of several other family members—but also with several medical problems of his own. During his interview, Benjamin indicates that he also sees Dorothy as a hero, because she has worked so hard at her recovery and has kept such a positive attitude.

Dorothy and Benjamin have allowed the experience of the stroke to deepen their relationship. They were newlyweds when Dorothy had her stroke and had only just begun to get adjusted to each other. Through the experience of the stroke, they have grown closer. They have learned how to share their feelings and work through misunderstandings. They are honest about how difficult this has been but have been able to maintain a positive attitude. Dorothy's recovery has been something they have worked on together, which has enriched their relationship. They have also kept a sense of humor with each other and are grateful to have each other's help.

For Benjamin, the experience of taking care of Dorothy has had several major, positive impacts. First, this experience has forced him to learn quickly that he is no longer number one in the house. He does several new chores—such as cooking and cleaning—that he had never done before. He admits to getting tired of this but does not seem to hold any resentment. Ben's traditional male upbringing and the perspectives that accompany this upbringing were an initial hindrance for him as a caregiver. It wasn't "natural" for him to cook, clean, or care for someone who is sick. However, he has undertaken it all and seems to have grown through this experience. Since he is retired but still physically healthy (most of the time), he has had the necessary time to be a caregiver.

Benjamin explains how the neurosurgeon told him that he and Dorothy needed to decide whether they wanted to prepare for the convalescent home or for coming home. If they chose for Dorothy to come home,
it would involve a tremendous amount of work. The neurosurgeon suggested they get Dorothy all the physical therapy they could. Ben said
the main goal had always been for her to come home, and they worked
hard toward this. It seems that by keeping this goal in front of them,
they kept up their spirits and became more flexible regarding traditional
gender roles. Ben looks for ways to have Dorothy practice her skills—
such as calling relatives on the phone or ordering from a menu at a
restaurant. Dorothy expressed gratitude to Ben for all the progress she
has made. Both of them seem to have accepted the challenge and worked
toward recovery.

Patricia has taken on many new responsibilities, which she identifies primarily as a loss in her life. In addition to taking care of Otto,
she has had to assume more responsibility for running their household.
Otto used to handle all the finances, plus help her around the house.
Now Patricia has to do it all. She says she struggles with keeping their
finances in order, but she admits she enjoys having more control. Formerly, Otto was the head of the household—typical of most traditional
marriages of their era. He earned the living and made the major decisions. Patricia was housewife and mother. Now the roles are reversed.
Despite experiencing the new responsibilities as a loss, Patricia feels
self-confident and energized. Otto feels worthless and depressed. She
is doing a fairly good job of handling the situation; he isn't doing so well.

Patricia has been successful in part because she receives emotional
support from her family and friends. Some of her friends can empathize
with her since they have had to deal with similar situations. Her family helps her take care of Otto. They come to visit or sit with him when
Patricia wants to go out in the evenings. Patricia is more fortunate than
many caregivers in this regard. Even with this support, it should be
noted that she often feels guilty about leaving Otto at home. Thus,
even with family support, Patricia, like most wives and husbands, feels
that she should be the primary caregiver. Family and friends can be
helpful but are rarely a substitute for a spouse. Perhaps her family and

friends could provide support by coming over to her house when she is home—not just when she wants to get out. This way she could stay home and feel less guilty, yet still have a bit more freedom from constantly having to attend to Otto's needs.

Though coping in a fairly effective way with the dramatic changes in her life, Patricia has experienced a loss of freedom and at times misses the role she once had in her marriage as housewife and mother. Prior to Otto's stroke, she had a fairly active social life. She bowled twice a week, went to a nearby resort once a month, and was active in her church. She misses all of this but has chosen to remain optimistic and positive about her situation. She knows that one day she will not be able to care for Otto by herself. Until then, she will continue to be his primary caregiver.

Like many caregivers, Patricia is responsible for giving and monitoring her husband's medications. In addition to his high blood pressure medication, Otto takes medications for depression and gout. He was given Prozac when he started having crying episodes. Clearly, as Patricia noted during her individual interview, Otto's behavior has changed dramatically since his stroke. Like many male stroke survivors, he is now more likely to cry (hence he is taking antidepressants). Yet this tendency to cry may be less a case of depression than of newly emerging freedom to express feelings, for Otto is also much more openly affectionate with Patricia than he ever was prior to the stroke. He tells her he loves her and indicates that he wants to resume a sexual relationship with her. Patricia is not quite sure how to handle the "new Otto."

Betty is also not sure how to handle her "new John." The ambivalence that Patricia experienced was echoed by Betty, who has noticed a significant change in John's personality since his stroke. In many ways, she likes him better since his stroke. Like Otto, he is now more inclined to talk about his feelings and is less demanding and kinder. He is more considerate of her feelings and seems "mellower." Betty also mentioned, as did Patricia, that she is becoming the "man" in her family, since she is the one now who carries the groceries, cleans the rain gutters, and generally does the heavy work that John used to do around the house. At times she feels a little trapped and senses that she has lost some control over her life. In other ways, she feels like she has gained more control with regard to her home and their finances.

Patricia reported feeling guilty when she leaves her husband to be taken care of by other members of the family. Betty also feels guilt, but in her case, the guilt arises when she gets impatient with John because he has been very demanding of her attention. She states that it's "like having a different person at home," and at times she misses the security of having a "strong man" around. Betty doesn't miss the more critical aspects of his personality that seem to have departed following the stroke but feels that she has had to "bury the former John" and went through a time of mourning for the man she knew intimately for many years.

Like many caregivers, Patricia is in the process of constructing a new image of her loved one. Much as stroke survivors must often recreate their physical and psychological selves after the stroke, so must the caregivers recreate their images of this new person and adjust their expectations about, their relationship with, and even their emotions in response to the stroke survivor. Change of this magnitude is a major task for anyone and in these cases is compounded by the grieving that inevitably takes place when bidding farewell to the old person and becoming acquainted with the new person.

In some ways, Patricia and Betty, like many of the women we interviewed, greatly appreciate and often feel flattered by the new emotional and even sexual attention they are getting from their husbands. Yet this new attention comes at a price, for their husbands often cry much more than they used to and frequently become more dependent and even childlike in their relationships with their wives. In many instances, female caregivers report that they have replaced one set of children (their "real" children) with another child (their husband). Like Betty, they have had to bury and mourn their former husbands, while taking some joy in the more emotional husbands with whom they are now living.

Bea finds some of the same gains and losses as Patricia, Betty, and many of the other female caregivers. She believes that she has gained several things from Ted's stroke that she hadn't anticipated. First, she has become much more involved in family decision making. Also, she is now reading to Ted. She wasn't one to read much before Ted had his stroke, but now she reads the newspaper to Ted for two hours in the morning before breakfast and two hours in the evening before going to bed. Needless to say, she is much more aware of what is going on in the world.

In general, being a caregiver to Ted is not a particular problem for Bea. She does what she has to and perceives that there are few losses. The one potentially problematic area concerns interpersonal relationships. The "ripple effect" for friends and family has been considerable. Bea mentioned that they aren't invited many places anymore by either family or friends. People come across as though they aren't sure of themselves when they're with Bea and Ted. Former friends seem a bit "standoffish." This doesn't bother Bea or Ted particularly, for they would have a hard time reciprocating anyway. Individually, Bea is no longer called to do things, largely because she has had to turn down the invitations of family and friends too many times. She is not comfortable leaving Ted.

A second potential loss for Bea and Ted concerns their inability to travel. Since his stroke, Ted has often been unable to remember recent trips that they have taken together. But he does remember those that took place twenty years ago and mentions them over and over again. Bea is accepting and patient, which Ted greatly appreciates. They don't go on as many trips as they used to. Ted loved to take trips; however, Bea feels relieved, in that she has arthritis and can't do as much as she used to. During the few trips they do take, Bea and Ted always help each other out. Bea is glad that their energy levels are more balanced now.

For Mary and Ralph, the inability to travel is definitely a loss. Like Bea and Ted, Mary and Ralph used to travel a great deal and often were quite spontaneous in deciding to take a trip. They also enjoyed taking courses together. With a considerable sense of frustration, Mary indicated that Ralph's stroke has led to closure in their life that is like being on a circular treadmill. The most exciting thing in their life, according to Mary, is "waiting for the garbage truck." She said that Ralph seems like a different person since his stroke. Because of extensive brain damage, he now speaks in a monotone and tires easily. His short-term memory is also poor, and he finds it difficult to process information. As a result, he gets confused when watching television. The changes in his physical strength have been more subtle. Mary constantly attempts to find new challenges for Ralph, so that he doesn't become complacent or give up hope. At present, he can walk one block. She is trying to get him to walk that second block.

Mary began to weep when discussing these limitations in her life. She attributed her weeping spells to the medication she is taking and denied that she is sad. It is readily apparent that psychological counseling would be advantageous for her and perhaps for Ralph as well. At the present time, Mary is afraid that if she phoned other caregivers, she would talk about Ralph's stroke all the time. Her level of tension and frustration suggests that she needs an outlet and some outside support. Mary's role, like the role played by many other female caregivers, has shifted from wife to mother.

Much like an attentive mother, Mary is providing cognitive stimulation for her husband. She is also nurturing autonomy and preparing Ralph for self-sufficiency. He is taking his own steps toward autonomy, in his woodworking and in his own "adolescent" rebellion from Mary's control (for example, wanting to take the car out without her knowledge). When asked about her contributions to Ralph's recovery, Mary cited her advocacy and her determination to continue supporting him, even when progress is slow. But what about her? Where does she find support and encouragement? Where does she find cognitive stimulation and new, personally gratifying challenges in her life?

Sylvia was more conscious than Mary of the problems she confronts and the losses she has experienced in taking care of Steven. Yet there were inconsistencies in many of her comments. On the one hand, she indicated that she enjoys the new role of being the primary decision maker in her family: "I enjoy this role for a change, because [Steven] always dictated to me and my children." Then in her next statement, she observed that "I am so nervous about this tax evaluation. I don't know where to begin. I have never done it [she recently received a letter from the IRS requesting an audit], and this letter from the insurance company—I don't know what to do with it." Sylvia was obviously anxious during her interview and often burst into tears. She stated that she could benefit most from a person who could advise or direct her in financial matters, including insurance papers and tax audits. All in all, Sylvia had never addressed the psychological aspects of her adjustment to Steven's stroke. She said she had never thought about this subject; no one had ever suggested that she receive professional counseling or attend a support group.

Although most of Sylvia's friends have maintained their close relationship with her and have shown appreciative sympathy, a few have upset her with comments such as: "How can anyone take a person like him to a restaurant?" Sylvia is still going through the grieving process. Her anger and resentment contrast with the deep sadness that envelops Steven. She feels that Steven's stroke could have been prevented if more registered nurses had been available to take care of him while he was in the intensive care unit following his coronary artery bypass surgery. The stroke occurred while nursing assistants were helping him to move from a chair to his bed. Sylvia believes that the hospital staff "forced him to move out of the intensive care unit too soon and the aides didn't know what they were doing." However, she is trying to rationalize the situation by saying, "There is a reason for everything. There must be a reason for this, too."

For sixty-six years, Sylvia's world was home, children, and Steven. Yet no one recognized her emotional turmoil and stress enough to suggest professional counseling. The interview provided her with a chance to speak with an empathic listener for the first time. However, listening is not enough. As Sylvia (and Steven) freely expressed their feelings and concerns, the interviewer became painfully aware of Sylvia's need for more support. Her church group provided invaluable early support, and her prayers have been a source of comfort and guidance. Yet she needs more than this; like many caregivers, she should be encouraged to find professional help during this particularly difficult life transition.

Lessons Learned by the Caregivers

Caregivers have not only experienced gains and losses; they have also learned something about the process of rehabilitation and about the most appropriate role they can play in this process. Hopefully the lessons they have learned can help other caregivers maximize the gains and minimize the losses. When asked to reflect on her own experiences as a caregiver, Karen indicates that she doesn't try to "make sense of the stroke" but does recommend that caregivers not "waste time being bitter about their fate." Since she retired early this year, she has been going to her husband's support group and has heard a lot of "living in the past" and complaints about "why did this happen to us?" Both Karen and Derrin acknowledge a deep need for each other. He needs her to take care of him and encourage him; she needs him as a companion—someone to care about and care for. The most important thing for Karen is that Derrin is still with her. Karen realizes that many of her widowed friends would be grateful to have a husband who had a stroke. At least she still has a husband.

Bea would tell other caregivers that the best way to adapt to and help other people cope with the aftermath of a stroke is to be patient and keep as healthy as possible. Also, caregivers shouldn't try to do too much, or they might get too tired. Bea claimed that she was not in need of financial, interpersonal, psychological, or physical services during the poststroke recovery period. She urges caregivers to be optimistic. Progress reports from the doctor are important, for they often show subtle improvement. Things do get better. Bea suggested that caregivers never give up trying to do fun things together with the stroke survivor and focus on the things they can easily do together.

When Benjamin was asked what he had learned from his experiences as a caregiver, he suggested that his most important insight concerned his willingness to get outside help. The critical decision for him was hiring a niece to come in daily to assist his wife with her exercises. He believes Dorothy worked much harder and made more progress because of the encouragement his niece provided. Having someone else to push Dorothy and stay on her to improve took the pressure off Benjamin. Dorothy was still in her wheelchair, but the doctor said she should be able to walk. So Ben told his niece that he would buy her a round-trip ticket to Europe if she could get Dorothy to walk. This motivator seemed to have worked, for Dorothy soon learned to walk! Ben sees this as the most important thing he has done in coping with her stroke.

Benjamin also learned something about finances and stroke rehabilitation. The most difficult adjustment for him has been the medical billing system. His biggest headache is straightening out the medical bills, and he would like to see this change for other caregivers. He encourages them to learn more about the billing system and to receive some help if needed (from friends, other family members, or outside services) to complete this difficult task.

Like Benjamin, Mary spoke of the need for stroke survivors to find stimulation in their lives, and like him, employed an outside person to provide this impetus. Mary's husband, Ralph, is a creative person who always loved working in his backyard shop. She has arranged for him to work on projects—including a bird feeder and a dictionary stand—in his workshop. This has been facilitated by two-hour visits twice a week by a student aide from the local community college. The student is enthusiastic because he has always wanted to learn how to use tools. In this way, Ralph not only receives the support and encouragement he needs but also has an opportunity to feel like he is of value to another person, since he is teaching the student about woodwork. The student not only encourages Ralph; his being there gives Mary the free time to pursue a painting class she enjoys. A year ago, Mary bought Ralph a reading stand and reading glasses. This is an added source of stimulation. He enjoys reading for several hours at a time and has read two or three novels during the year, usually action-based books about planes, war, cowboys, or the Navy. In this way, Ralph has been able to displace and reduce some of his frustration regarding lack of strength and control.

Leonard also found outside help to be invaluable for him as a caregiver to Kevin. Leonard noted that when Kevin came home from the hospital, he posed quite a challenge: "After about ten days I took him home. The first day home was terrifying. He had a wheelchair, he could walk, but he refused. I told him that he would have to get up and go to the bathroom on his own. I just couldn't continue to do that. . . . A social worker came by a lot the first couple of weeks. It really helped me to not feel so trapped. I didn't know if I could trust Kevin by himself and he was terrified that something might happen to him when I was not here."

Learning from Family Caregivers 217

Thus, the outside support not only helped Leonard feel less confined by the caregiving role but also provided assurance to Kevin that someone would always be there to help out. In addition, the outside assistance helped Leonard get his energy back so that he could continue with the demanding job of Kevin's rehabilitation: "Getting around [is] the most difficult aspect of the stroke. . . . It takes an overwhelming physical effort [for the caregiver as well as stroke survivor]. You get so tired. . . . I have to keep pushing Kevin or he will not do anything. [I must] keep him moving. . . . [It is] exasperating work."

When asked what advice he would give other caregivers, Leonard suggested that caregivers get time away, "because otherwise it gets to be too much. . . . Make life as normal as possible for everyone. Do not treat them as if they were an invalid. Help them to become independent, both mentally and physically." He wished that there were support groups exclusively for people who are taking care of stroke survivors: "You need to take time off so you can change your focus of attention. Otherwise our personal world is 'too much for us,' as someone said. . . . It is really hard work. Sometimes you can't see the light at the end of the tunnel. It's important to see other people and other faces."

The lessons that Patricia learned as a caregiver were identical to several already noted: taking care of oneself and getting extra help, whenever possible, from friends, family, and professionals. Like most other caregivers, she feels that the caregiving role is demanding and that it is important to prepare for even worse conditions, if the health of the survivor should deteriorate. Unlike many of the other caregivers, however, Patricia goes beyond the immediate caregiving situation and suggests that outside assistance is necessary not only for her own welfare, but also for the welfare of the person she is caring for. She wonders what she will do if her husband's condition gets worse. Physically, she realizes that she is limited in the amount of care she can provide, and she is starting to look for alternatives in the event this happens.

This crucial lesson is often overlooked by caregivers. They may eventually be successful in adjusting to the demands of their stroke survivor's disabilities, but they often fail to anticipate changes in these conditions.

They may be looking forward to and have planned for the day when their loved one gets better and no longer needs as much assistance. However, they often practice denial when it comes to the equally great possibility that their loved one could have another stroke or could decline in terms of either physical health or willingness to confront physical and emotional problems. As Patricia noted, it is critical that caregivers take care of themselves and obtain outside assistance; otherwise, they will never be able to cope with any worsening problems.

Betty reiterated the importance of both self-care and support. She emphasized the value of a support group, not only as a source of emotional support but also as a source of information and a vehicle for sharing experiences. She felt lucky that John's stroke had not disabled him nearly as much as many other men and women who have had strokes. She became aware of this fact by attending a stroke support group. The perspectives she has gained from this group have been invaluable. Comparing her experiences with those of other caregivers, Betty has grown to appreciate the ways John has accepted his stroke. He seems not to be fighting the rehabilitation and has not become bitter. In growing to appreciate his strength, Betty is more accepting of her own role as caregiver.

Other caregivers also commented on the value of support groups for them, several of the people we interviewed suggesting that caregivers have their own support group. Tina reiterated Betty's sense that a stroke support group can be a wonderful place to talk with other caregivers and stroke survivors who have gone through similar experiences. Tina found that the support group also helped to reduce some of her resentment about the lack of empathy and assistance that she was getting from others: "It is so important to have people who listen and understand." For her, going to the stroke support group was a cleansing and healing experience. It enabled her to resolve many of her feelings about other people in her life and to begin establishing a better relationship with them. As a result, she has been able to ask for help more directly from these friends and relatives. At first she couldn't see how she could find time for the support group, but now she believes that it is more important for both Parker and herself than any of the physical therapy or checkups he receives.

Adding further to her list of lessons learned, Betty agrees with Patricia that finding time for oneself is critical as a caregiver. Betty indicated that being with John at home all the time requires that she find some space and time for herself. She accomplishes this by walking alone for five to seven miles a day. She also regularly walks with John (in conjunction with his rehabilitation), as a way of linking her own free-time activities with the activities she shares with him.

Betty added another lesson learned to the brief list that Patricia provided. She said she had learned a particularly difficult lesson: caregivers cannot do everything for the stroke survivor; they must allow their loved one to struggle with certain tasks and responsibilities and accomplish them on their own. Throughout this book, we have talked about the need to balance support and challenge. Betty is pointing directly to this issue. If caregivers try to do everything for the stroke survivor, they are likely to be unsuccessful, especially if they are themselves incapable of being highly active because of age or their own physical problems. More important, they also are preventing the stroke survivor from reestablishing a sense of identity and self-worth.

Betty mentioned that while it hurts her to see her husband struggle and she is often frustrated by his slow progress, his rehabilitation has brought the two of them closer as they face the task of recovery together. He is more open in expressing his emotions and more willing to communicate, in part because he needs to work closely with Betty, rather than working by himself or letting her do everything for him. The newfound interdependence between Betty and John has enhanced their own relationship, as many other long-married couples also reported. Furthermore, the recovery process has provided new challenges for Betty (and other caregivers).

With sufficient support from family, friends, professionals, and her husband, Betty can meet these new challenges. She learned that she can handle her new situation and has found that she can do things she never thought were in her grasp. Dan similarly suggests that "I learned I had a great capacity to do more things for my mother than I thought I could . . . to handle household chores without feeling bitter about it." He suggests that "most of all, what [stroke survivors] need is a lot of

love, a lot of little hugs, and a lot of 'everything's going to be all right.'"
He has discovered that he can give this to his mother. He has also discovered, however, that after having already lost a father and two brothers
and having supported his mother through three strokes, he also needs
this love and assurance that "everything's going to be all right."

Such is the way of human maturation and learning. Both challenge
and support must be present for either to occur. Caregivers can gain
much from the challenge of taking care of a loved one. Their own values
in life and their own sense of purpose and self-worth can be enhanced.
However, this will only occur if they receive love and support from
those around them who concern themselves with the welfare and rehabilitation of both the stroke survivor and the caregivers. As many
of the caregivers we interviewed noted, their relationship with the stroke
survivor is often complex and emotionally charged. At some point soon
after the stroke, most caregivers experience a sense of guilt, either because in some way they feel they could have helped their loved one
prevent the stroke in the first place or because they feel they are not
doing enough to help the survivor with the rehabilitation. They feel
negligent or helpless.

Neither of these feelings is of much value in the recovery process.
As Shimberg (1990, p. 13), herself a caregiver, has noted: "Never feel
guilty for whatever you're thinking. Strokes don't happen in a vacuum.
They not only affect the person who suffers the stroke, but they also
upset the balance of the entire family. Your life changed with the stroke
too. There's no use pretending that things will be the same. They won't.
They can't. You have a right to wonder how you'll be affected. All your
so-called wild thoughts are normal ones under the circumstances. I've
had them. Everyone who's loved a stroke survivor has too." As we turn
in the final two chapters to the perspectives offered by a professional
caregiver, we will see this important theme repeatedly stated: caregivers
must take care of themselves and act on behalf of their own welfare
and feelings, not just those that are assumed to belong to the survivor.
Erich Fromm (1956) has suggested that we can't truly love others until
we have learned to love ourselves. Similarly, we can't effectively care
for others until we have learned to care for ourselves.

14

On Being a Professional Helper

I (Barbara Kobylinski) am a clinical social worker at an outpatient rehabilitation center. Working with the survivors of stroke is a challenge and a privilege. Sometimes it is a joyful experience and sometimes a sad experience. When I first entered the field, I was already familiar with caregiving, having been a wife and mother for many years. However, I was now counseling stroke survivors and their families and had been placed in charge of leading a stroke support group. I was apprehensive at first and wondered if my clinical skills would be appropriate in helping these men and women grieve for the loss of their past life and the skills they so readily employed during their prestroke years. Could I successfully help these people empower themselves to invest in a different life-style, accept their limitations, and learn to work within them? I was now on a journey of learning, healing, and growing within myself and with the survivors of strokes and their families.

Rehabilitation Center

Most stroke survivors go from an acute inpatient hospital setting to some form of outpatient rehabilitation service. Some survivors receive home health services, which include nursing care (when appropriate), occupational therapy, physical therapy, and speech therapy. When survivors can tolerate two to three hours of therapy two or three times per week, they can be referred by their doctor to an outpatient rehabilitation center.

At an outpatient rehab center, health professionals usually work as a team. As the social worker, I saw all survivors who had at least two or three weekly sessions scheduled in occupational, physical, or speech therapy. I completed an interview with the survivors and their families called a *psychosocial assessment*. This assessment enabled me to evaluate the survivors' adjustment and the type of support available from family members. This information helps the other therapists understand the family dynamics. These findings were discussed at bimonthly team sessions involving myself and the occupational, physical, and speech therapists.

After the survivors have been treated at the outpatient rehab center for at least one month, they can join the stroke support group. Some doctors choose home health services for stroke survivors due to their nursing needs at the time of their discharge from an inpatient acute setting. Occasionally, some stroke survivors do not continue on to an outpatient rehab center. These survivors can become isolated at home due to the absence of interaction with other stroke survivors. They lack the socialization and support they could receive through attending the support group.

Stroke Support Group

Typically, the stroke support group at an outpatient rehab center constitutes the primary group counseling program for stroke survivors and their families. This is a structured group, sometimes informal, where people can share their experiences in a supportive atmosphere. Typically, the overall goal is to help survivors and families meet their emotional and educational needs. The objectives are to encourage a positive attitude and to help survivors make life-style adjustments after the stroke. In addition, the support group offers a social opportunity for survivors and families to share their experiences under the guidance of a professional. At the outpatient rehab center where I worked, this group typically consisted of eight to twenty members and met once a week to maintain a sense of community.

My first support group consisted of survivors who had had strokes anywhere from three months to eleven years earlier as well as their caregivers (mostly spouses and adult children). The members attending the group were 40 percent from the outpatient program and 60 percent from among those who were either discharged survivors or their families. I have always enjoyed leading groups, but this was a truly unique group—the most challenging group I have ever led. It was a challenge for me because the survivors in this particular group were faced with another loss after their stroke. They had been led by another social worker from an inpatient program for over a year. It was difficult for the members to accept this change and acknowledge me as their new friend and group leader. My work had just begun.

At the beginning of this first support group experience, I used a video to explain strokes and to help educate the survivors and their families about warning signs, risk factors, and different types of strokes. Some survivors remembered how their stroke happened. Others were unable to recall anything about the experience. As is often the case— and as we have documented throughout this book—most survivors were not knowledgeable about their stroke. They did not know the proper names for the different types of strokes—such as *embolic, thrombotic, hemorrhagic,* or *lacunar*—or what type they had experienced. Some survivors were fearful about asking physicians about changing medications or reducing the amounts of medication they were taking. After establishing a basic understanding of the risks, warning signs, and types of strokes, we invited a neurologist to give a presentation on various aspects of strokes and to answer questions from the group.

Trina was a survivor and a member of the first support group I led. She had suffered a mild stroke, which resulted in minor weakness in her left hand. She remembered that this particular neurologist had treated her in the hospital. She did not, however, remember what type of stroke she had suffered and now had a chance to ask him. It had been about six months since her stroke had occurred. She raised her hand excitedly and asked what specific type of stroke she had suffered. The neurologist stated that she had suffered a lacunar stroke. She was elated to finally know exactly what had occurred and why she was able to recover so quickly.

The doctor told the group that he does try to explain exactly what type of stroke has occurred, and the process for healing and recovery, to all his patients and their families while the survivors are hospitalized. But he said that many families and survivors are in the stages of shock and denial just after the stroke has occurred and so do not hear the information given to them at the hospital. He tries to follow up with most of his patients but is not always able to reach them. This issue of survivors and caregivers receiving timely information was certainly an important theme for most of the people we interviewed for this book, and I have found this to be a critical issue among the survivors I see at the outpatient rehab center as well.

Trina stayed in the support group for only four weeks. She had difficulty relating to the other survivors. Her stroke was minor and left her with only slight impairment in her left hand. She wanted desperately to recover 100 percent. When she saw the other members in the group with severe limitations, she struggled with reaching her goal of total recovery. As it turned out, she did not recover completely but learned to accept her slight limitations and continued to travel in her recreational vehicle with her husband. She eventually passed her driver's license test and felt good about her accomplishments. She had learned to establish goals in her life again and achieve them.

Another aspect of coping with a stroke is learning good nutrition and understanding the importance of using medications to prevent future strokes. A nutritionist from the hospital gave a presentation on eating properly and planning a nutritious diet and explained how to cope with the challenge of the swallowing reflex. A pharmacist was then invited to identify the different types of medication taken for hypertension, such as blood thinners and aspirin. A few group members were diabetic and needed information on how the different medications interacted with their current medications and could produce adverse reactions.

Another area discussed was medication that caused mood changes. The survivors had many questions about why they had to stay on certain types of medications and about the long-term effects of these medications. The pharmacist urged them to check with their primary doctor about any problems with medications; in particular, mood shifts or other changes in the survivor's condition should be reported. Maura, who had been in the group for two years, was concerned about the amount of medication she was taking and had never asked her doctor to change her prescriptions. She had been feeling fatigued for several weeks. After talking to the pharmacist, she made a commitment to urge her physician to change her medication or to at least ask the doctor to reevaluate her current needs. I was impressed with her willingness to be assertive and to get her needs met. It was also encouraging for me to see the changes she was making by being open.

Strokes frequently affect vision. Because of these visual changes, we asked an ophthalmologist to give a presentation concerning the impact of strokes on vision. Hemianopsia is the major visual impairment that can result from a stroke. This impairment results from damage to the optic nerve, leaving the stroke survivor blind in one half of each eye. The same half of each eye is affected corresponding to the side of the body that is affected. The ophthalmologist explained that therapy or glasses will not completely resolve this vision problem but that compensatory techniques can be learned.

Another type of impairment is called *one-sided neglect.* It is an unconscious perceptual impairment resulting in lack of awareness of the side of the body and environment on the affected side; if combined with hemianopsia, high potential for injury exists. Some survivors experience spatial relationship disturbances, blurred vision, and inability to read. The doctor recommended that the survivors wait up to six months to change their glasses prescription due to the continued healing process of the brain. I feel powerless when I am not able to offer hope to some survivors, knowing that they will not have clear enough vision to read again or do other tasks. Vision problems that cannot be corrected represent a great loss.

Pete was a member of the first support group who experienced one-sided neglect. He was able to see only shadows with one eye but had good vision with his other eye. He recounted to the group members how he cut his grass only on the left side of his lawn when he returned home from the hospital. He also has had difficulty reading the newspaper but alleviated this problem by moving the paper over to the left side so that he could read the entire page. He has successfully compensated to the right and is able to drive his car to the support group each week.

At this stage in the group experience, I was amazed at what an impact guest speakers from the medical field could have on survivors and their families. As we have noted throughout this book, medical professionals can play a critical role in helping to foster a stroke survivor's sense of optimism and control. The group members had someone else to advocate for them and encourage them to live life to the fullest.

Once a month, the occupational, physical, and speech therapists gave presentations to the group that highlighted up-to-date information and current trends in their fields. The occupational therapist put together presentations on leisure activities that allow survivors to resume a productive life as part of the community. Gardening was frequently mentioned by many of the survivors. They discovered that they could continue this type of activity but had to make adjustments due to the effects of the stroke. Often this included use of only one arm or hand or transferring to an outside chair to repot plants and do other outdoor activities. Sally was able to resume gardening simply by following the suggestions of the occupational therapist. She felt that this allowed her to be productive again, to pot and plant flowers as she had before her stroke. What a joy it was to see her feeling productive again and sharing her excitement with the other members of the group. She was on the way to rebuilding her self-esteem.

The physical therapy presentations updated the survivors' exercise routines. They were told how important consistent exercise was to their recovery. Even after outpatient rehab, the need to do daily exercises continues indefinitely for all survivors. Braces were sometimes recommended for muscle, bone, or joint problems. Without the brace, the disability could worsen. Exercise routines needed to be updated, as in the case of George. He was an athletic person before his stroke and had reached the maximum potential of his present exercise routine. He requested a reevaluation at the rehab center and was given a more aggressive exercise routine, which challenged him and hastened his recovery. Occasionally survivors regress or do not progress further in their recovery. Reevaluation is available to determine if more therapy or additional exercises are needed. I have felt elated to see survivors walk again after struggling through their rehab program. There is a great sense of fulfillment when one observes survivors taking charge of their activities and continuing to work within their limitations.

In the speech therapy presentations, survivors learned techniques for improving memory. They were also given information on communication impediments after a stroke. Emphasis was placed on effective communication techniques that aphasic stroke survivors could use. Limitations frequently encountered by stroke survivors are the inability to hold the phone receiver on the affected side or to speak on the phone. A phone company representative presented information on the types of adaptive equipment available to disabled people. The phone rep brought several types of special phone equipment, such as speakerphones, cordless phones, small headsets, phones with adaptive hearing parts, and special phones for the blind. Most of the survivors used these telephone services.

Ted was a survivor who was in a wheelchair; he was paralyzed on one side and had difficulty speaking. He indicated in the group that he was unable to answer the phone and write down a message with his affected hand. He also had difficulty getting to his desk phone within five rings. When he chose his adaptive phone equipment, he received a cordless phone and holster for his wheelchair and also a speakerphone. In fact, he called me from this phone to tell me how much this service had meant to him, since it allowed him to communicate with his family and friends. This particular survivor had had difficulty accepting help in the past. What a wonderful change the phone equipment made. His life became easier and less stressful. I felt moved by his phone call and sensed he was changing and growing in his recovery process.

Caregiver Group

After I had begun facilitating my first support group for stroke survivors, the family members of the survivors expressed interest in forming a caregiver group. As noted previously, caregivers often feel that they receive little support or understanding from other people with regard to their own life changes associated with the stroke. The group was set up to meet once a month without survivors. Spouses (both men and women) and adult children of the survivors participated in the group. I often work more with the families than with the survivors. This happens because, as we've seen in previous chapters, the families are usually grieving as much or more than the survivors.

The purpose of the group was to offer emotional support to the caregivers and to give them an opportunity to voice their frustrations, successes, and failures in a safe environment without their survivors present and with others who are in similar situations. They learn how to take better care of themselves and how to reduce the stress they encounter as caregivers.

My experiences in working with the caregiver group convinced me that the right of caregivers to live and find enjoyment in life needs greater recognition. Melanie indicated in a support group session that she would like to be alone more often without having to worry about the stroke survivor she cares for. During these cherished times, she would like to be able to do what she wants to do without feeling guilty. Yet she feels obligated to take care of her survivor at all times and does not realize that she has any rights.

I obtained a copy of the *Caregiver's Bill of Rights* (Alzheimer's Society, 1992). This bill of rights was very meaningful to the caregivers, who told me that in times of frustration and indecision, they would read it again and again. The rights it spells out are as follows:

I have the right to make mistakes and to be imperfect

I have the right to forgive myself and begin anew

I have the right to say no and not feel guilty or selfish

I have the right to relax

I have the right to let go of yesterday and embrace today

I have the right to enlist the cooperation of my family

I have the right to laugh and be happy

I have the right to arrange my own priorities

I have the right to take time for myself

I have the right to have my needs considered important
to others

I have the right to be free to do special things for myself

I have the right to take time off even if it costs money

I have the right to take charge

I have the right to make decisions when other family
members refuse to participate

I have the right to be self-preserving so that I can care
for others

One caregiver, Betty, placed her copy of the bill of rights on her refrigerator and read it daily. Previously, she had no idea that the caregiver had any rights. They became more meaningful to her, especially the right to be free and do things for herself, the right to take time off even if it cost money, and the right to take charge. She traveled by attending a wedding and going to her fiftieth class reunion. She arranged to have family members stay with her husband while she was away. This contributed to her self-esteem and sense of self-worth, and she realized that she could occasionally meet her own needs and feel good about doing this without guilt. This was a major breakthrough for this caregiver. I was elated when I was able to experience her blooming as a person again.

I also secured a copy of Schmall and Stiehl's *Coping with Caregiving: How to Manage Stress When Caring for Elderly Relatives* (1989) for the caregivers. During six sessions, the group learned who they were as caregivers and completed a quiz on the symptoms and causes of stress. They also learned strategies for managing their stress. They had to set realistic goals and expectations, establish limits, ask for and accept help, take care of themselves, and involve other people.

Greta identified herself as a martyr. She consistently refused help and was often exhausted and irritable. After these sessions, she realized it was okay to ask for help, call others in the group and share frustrations, and involve her family in the caregiving of her husband. Her continued growth helped others in the group risk changing their lifestyles, too. She had become an advocate for herself and others. I was truly amazed at her progress and was encouraged that the group dynamics were working for the good of the caregivers.

Caregivers need to learn to love themselves. A good place to start might be with Louise Hay's *Ten Steps to Loving Yourself* (1993). The principles she outlines are as follows:

1. *Stop all criticism:* Criticism never changes a thing. Refuse to criticize yourself. Accept yourself exactly as you are. Everybody changes. When you criticize yourself, your changes are negative. When you approve of yourself, your changes are positive.

2. *Don't scare yourself:* Stop terrorizing yourself with your thoughts. It's a dreadful way to live. Find a mental image that gives you pleasure (mine is yellow roses), and immediately switch your scary thought to a pleasure thought.

3. *Be gentle and kind and patient:* Be gentle with yourself. Be kind to yourself. Be patient with yourself as you learn the new ways of thinking. Treat yourself as you would someone you really loved.

4. *Be kind to your mind:* Self hatred is only hating your own thoughts. Don't hate yourself for having the thoughts. Gently change your thoughts.

5. *Praise yourself:* Criticism breaks down the inner spirit. Praise builds it up. Praise yourself as much as you can. Tell yourself how well you are doing with every little thing.

6. *Support yourself:* Find ways to support yourself. Reach out to friends and allow them to help you. It is being strong to ask for help when you need it.

7. *Be loving to your negatives:* Acknowledge that you created them to fulfill a need. Now you are finding new, positive ways to fulfill these needs. So lovingly release the old negative patterns.

8. *Take care of your body:* Learn about nutrition. What kind of fuel does your body need to have optimum energy and vitality? Learn about exercise. What kind of exercise can you enjoy? Cherish and revere the temple you live in.

9. *Mirror work:* Look into your eyes often. Express this growing sense of love you have for yourself. Forgive yourself looking into the mirror. Talk to your parents looking into the mirror. Forgive them too. At least once a day say: "I love you. I really love you!"

10. *Do it now:* Don't wait until you get well, or lose the weight, or get a new job, or the new relationship. Begin now—do the best you can.

Most of the caregivers were moved by these principles. They realized that they had difficulty praising themselves and had been plagued by feelings of guilt, especially when they had to leave their survivors alone. It was frustrating for me to see that many had little self-esteem and were tired and depressed. We went over the principles and discussed ones that gave the group members difficulty or challenged them. We talked about how they could use the principles in their own situation; I also found myself considering ways that I could apply them in my own life. I saw many changes in this support group over the next two years, as caregivers grew and changed, became more assertive, and learned to share their frustrations and minor successes and failures with the group.

As we also discovered in our interviews, many caregivers experience a profound role reversal. The male is often the survivor, and for many years he had been taking care of family bills and providing the income. Now the wife has to accept these responsibilities, and it may be devastating and overwhelming for her. Some—particularly older women—have never paid bills or written checks during their marriage. Some spouses have no idea what type of insurance they carry, or how much money they have in the bank or in retirement plans.

I have worked with some adult children who are responsible for their parents, but I work mostly with spouses. I think it is harder for adult children to deal with parents who have suffered strokes because they are in the process of raising their own children and are now faced with an additional demand. Taking on the responsibility of caring for their elderly parents is frustrating. Sometimes the parent-child relationship was difficult in the past. Sometimes there is verbal or physical abuse of the parent or even neglect. Adult children may not respond to the needs of the parent in the way the parent would like. The most difficult challenge for me is when I have to call Adult Protective Services to report an adult child who has been abusing or neglecting a parent. I dislike reporting abuse; however, I am a mandated reporter and must advocate for the survivors. This abuse of the elderly parent by adult children tends to happen in dysfunctional families with poor communication and disrespect for the parents.

On the other hand, many adult children fully participate in the caregiver role. Their role in life is to do everything for their parent, often causing them to lose respect in their immediate family. A member from the immediate family would call me and say, "My mother's doing everything for my grandmother and she's not home when I need her. What should I do?" I tell the adult child that they can't do everything for their survivor. They need to start taking care of themselves and their own family. But I also encourage the families of caregivers to become less dependent and to acknowledge the change in family roles that has been made necessary by the survivor's recovery efforts. Some adult children want to take care of their parents because they feel responsible or feel guilty about certain family relationships. These feelings are to be expected when there is a catastrophe such as a parent suffering a stroke. But sometimes it may be best for the adult children to hire outside help in order to ensure their own health and sanity.

Occasionally I work with a stroke survivor who has no support or caregiver. I become the caregiver—the person responsible for providing support, helping the survivor get to resources, looking into in-home supportive services, searching for a chore worker, or meeting other needs. I become the adult child in that family and take over the role of advocating for that survivor. This is a difficult role to assume. It takes a considerable amount of energy and drains me emotionally when I cannot place a survivor, or when the location they are currently living in is not the best placement for them. I become concerned and worried about that survivor's recovery process. I am also concerned about their transportation, emotional adjustment, loneliness, and eating habits.

Sometimes survivors without caregivers want me to take care of them. Most of the time I want to look after them and help them get their needs met, but I can't do that all the time, since it can become quite tiring. I have had to learn to release these survivors and help them feel empowered to do things on their own. I have to refer them to adult day-care centers, churches, and volunteer groups that do home visits and to groups that do daily reassurance calling. These community resources can meet many of the needs of survivors without caregivers and can lessen their sense of isolation.

Professional Caregiving

No matter what the caregiver situation, I am very enthusiastic with all of the stroke survivors I have encountered. I try to support them completely as their caregiver or friend. I let them know that I believe in them and in their goodness. They know I care about them, because I convey this to them through things like sending cards or giving hugs. I am always looking for that glimmer of hope, that light within the survivors that will help them reinvest in their changed lives. But some survivors do not seem to get enough encouragement from their family. Sometimes I hear that relatives are disgusted or discouraged with them.

It's not easy to care for someone else 100 percent of the time. I encourage family members to negotiate and compromise with each other and to work out schedules so that everyone does their share.

A typical question that comes up during a caregiver group session is, "What will I do if my spouse dies?" My answer is that they will do the best they can under the circumstances. The caregiver group as well as family and friends can provide support. Also, there are many bereavement groups in the community through the hospitals and churches. I encourage caregivers to look within for inner strength and to look outside themselves for support from their family and church (where appropriate) to give them help and guidance. The odds of their spouses dying before them are great. But some caregivers who feel excessively stressed and do not accept enough outside help may precede their survivor in death. Then someone would be needed to take care of the survivor. These group sessions are frightening to most of the caregivers because they are faced with the reality of life and death.

15

Healing and
Letting Go

As a professional caregiver, I (Barbara Kobylinski) have come to realize that even though someone has had a stroke or is taking care of a stroke survivor, there are many different ways to heal and to grieve the loss of capacities or even of life. Survivors may not have a complete physical healing, but they can have an emotional, spiritual, or relationship healing. They can heal their relationship with God or some other divine presence in their life, or make changes to heal an area in their lives where they have difficulty. They can ask for forgiveness and find ways to release old, inadequate elements of their own life or relationships with other significant people.

Healing

In stroke support groups, we have discussed several different modes of healing. Sometimes we use meditation or guided imagery to achieve these goals. There are different ways to acknowledge healing within a person. Survivors can accept their limitations and make a choice that they are going to have a good quality of life. They can do this if they keep a positive attitude. I think that when people have suffered a stroke, everything comes to a sudden stop. They get a chance to look at what they have done in the past, where they are now, and where the future may lead them. The unknown aspect of the future seems especially difficult for these survivors to cope with. They may have only five years to live or maybe twenty, but they have to make a choice about how they are going to live. They can live within their limitations.

Some survivors do not look or feel the way they did before their stroke. They can work through these feelings of grief and loss and still feel good about who they are as human beings. I try to accept these people where they are. Some may be in denial, some are depressed, and some are able to accept their limitations. Most have the expectation of 100 percent return in their arms and legs, but this does not happen often. They all deserve to have a good quality of life and a sense of dignity and value. The majority of survivors that I have worked with have chosen to grow and change, but the process has been painful and difficult for them. Most survivors have learned to be patient and persevere with encouragement, caring, and love from family, friends, and the rehab team.

Stroke survivors go through many of the same stages of grieving as terminally ill patients. These stages were first described by Elisabeth Kübler-Ross in her book *On Death and Dying* (1969). These stages are denial and isolation, anger, bargaining, depression, and acceptance. The families of survivors go through the same stages of grieving. Most people go in and out of the stages at different times, not necessarily in the order stated above. Since the survivor is rarely in the same stage as the caregiver, it is hard for empathy to occur on the part of the family members.

Two of the most difficult stages for survivors and their families are denial and depression. As we have noted elsewhere in this book, there is a place for denial in the healing process. Denial provides a safe place in which to gain strength before looking at reality. But when people have been in denial at the rehabilitation center for two or three months and can't move forward, this must be addressed. I share my feelings with the survivors and confront them where they are stuck. I realize it is difficult and painful for them, but at some point they have to make the leap. They have to face reality.

Some stroke survivors don't want a healthy dose of reality, since they sometimes find reality distressing. They may not use the arm or hand to play ball, knit, or cook the way they did before. It's such a great loss for some survivors. They become disillusioned in their denial. We can't promise them full recovery because every stroke is unique and every person is unique. Return of function depends on what area of the brain has been affected and how severe that damage is. When survivors see other people in the gym progressing faster than they are, it's difficult to explain that the process is different for everyone. I continually encourage survivors to focus on their own unique recovery process. I support them in acknowledging their achievements and celebrating their successes.

A good example of denial occurred with one particular survivor, Marco. He would not talk about anything from the past because it made him feel very emotional, and he had never been a feeling person. Since he had suffered a stroke, he had become quite emotional and cried whenever I mentioned the past or his family. He refused to come and discuss these feelings with me. He told me he thought I was a nosy social worker. I was trying to get him to realize that by talking about painful things from the past, he could resolve some of the issues that were blocking his progress. He was unable to accept the challenge. He could not understand that by holding on to old negative feelings, he was blocking his movement toward healing and recovery. He could not accept that. He could not talk with me or open up to the expression of his grief. His family came to me for help in dealing with this situation and asked me for ways to assist them. There was nothing I could do but accept this survivor and support him at this particular crossroad in his life. He chose denial, and nothing I could do or say would change the essential character of this person.

Depression is commonly experienced by both survivors and caregivers, It is a natural part of the grieving process. We discuss depression and the warning signs of depression in our support groups. Hopelessness, helplessness, and fatigue are common characteristics of depression. During the support group, we also consider the role that physical exhaustion plays in causing or exacerbating depression. Physical demands such as interrupted sleep and lack of healthy exercise are commonly associated with depression. We examine ways to deal with the depression, and I suggest ways the survivors and caregivers can change their behavior to improve their self-image, increase their sense of self-worth, and build on any optimism they might hold at some level. Goal setting and time structuring help to alleviate depression. We also talk about cases where the survivor is depressed over an extended period of time and may need counseling or antidepressant medication prescribed by their doctor or psychiatrist. Some of the group members typically express apprehension about the use of medication. I try to assure them that their doctor might recommend short-term use of medicines that can be quite beneficial. Many survivors were pessimistic before their stroke and are now even more negative. This sometimes contributes further to the depressive state of some caregivers.

Death is frequently on the mind of the caregiver. Typically, the members of a caregiver support group discuss how they would react to the loss of their survivor and what stages of grief they would go through. About midyear in my first year of group facilitation, one of the survivors (Bert) learned he was diagnosed with stomach cancer. It was at an inoperable stage. His mother had died from this type of cancer and his wife (Janice), fearing the worst, discussed her frightened feelings in the caregiver group. I decided to work with Bert and Janice and continued up to the time of his death. During the six weeks before his death, Bert listened to Bernie Siegel tapes (Siegel, 1990a) and read his book *Peace, Love, and Healing* (Siegel, 1990b). We discussed his feelings about dying. He was not afraid to die and was busy reading and calling old friends and making amends with people. His daughters had come to visit and help take care of him for a few weeks. He was weak but coping with his pain.

There was only one area he wanted to clear up before he died. He desperately wanted his wife to forgive him for some old wounds that were not healed from the past. I discussed these wishes with her, but she was not ready to respect his wishes or to forgive him. I told her when the time came she would be ready and just to think about what a healing this would be for both of them. I left their house feeling angry and upset and cried all the way home. This man had progressed so much and invested in life. He had given a presentation on strokes for the stroke support group. He had progressed and, damn it, it was not fair for him to die. I felt unsettled with his wife's decision to not forgive him; I hoped she could let him die with dignity and peace.

I felt a large amount of emotion exploding inside me when I got home, displaced my anger at my husband, and was emotionally drained for the rest of the evening. I thought to myself, I am not getting close to any more survivors or caregivers again. It's just too painful. My husband, thank God, was understanding and supportive as I went through my own grieving process. My client died two days later. His wife called to tell me that she had a change of heart the evening before he died and had forgiven the wounds of the past, which made him happy and peaceful. Miracles do happen and healing does take place in many ways. I feel privileged to have been a witness to this healing.

I think it is very important for survivors to have something to believe in, whether it be a higher power, God, Buddha, or something that helps them during the times when they have no answers and have no one to turn to. It helps them feel empowered and motivated to persevere in adjusting to their new life. I build rapport and trust with survivors and their families before I feel comfortable asking questions about their spirituality. It's not a common question you ask while conducting an interview or writing an assessment. After survivors and their caregivers get to know me and trust me, I feel comfortable asking questions about religion, meaning in life, and death and dying. For many survivors, spirituality is an integral part of their recovery process.

Some survivors have shared their experiences with me. A member of our stroke support group, Jose, had a heart attack during a meeting. It was a frightening scene for some of the members. The main questions asked were, "Did he have another stroke?" and "Is he going to die?" Fortunately, he did not die. He was taken to the hospital via ambulance and recovered. His wife later disclosed in their support group that if it had not been for their faith in God and his goodness, Jose might have died. The subject of spirituality does come up during the support group meetings. Some members have indicated that after they had their stroke, their belief in a higher power increased and became more intimate. This belief gave them the courage and perseverance to continue with life. For some members, though, belief in God or some other higher power decreased after their stroke, as a result of the anger and frustration associated with their loss.

Sex is a difficult subject for most survivors in a support group to discuss. Caregivers, however, often want to "compare notes" and find out how they can get their sexual needs met again. There is not enough in the literature about sex after strokes, but the National Stroke Association newsletter *Be Stroke Smart* (Glass, 1990) contains some useful articles. They answer many of the questions caregivers have regarding when to resume sex, if sexual activity is likely to cause another stroke, and if age has any bearing on resuming sex. Sexual dysfunction is a common problem of stroke survivors, and physical disabilities sometimes preclude sex.

Many caregivers are fearful about even suggesting a sexual encounter with their partner after the stroke. Most survivors are afraid that they will have another stroke if they are sexually active. We describe several different positions the caregivers can try depending on the physical condition of their survivor. We also discuss different ways of being intimate without intercourse, including cuddling, kissing, manipulation, or just the simple act of tender touching and massage. Some caregivers are reticent about bringing up the topic of sexuality with their survivor's doctor or even with their spouse unless he or she asks for a sexual encounter. The change in the survivor's physical appearance is a factor that may cause the partner to no longer feel the sexual attraction that had been present in their earlier relationship.

Another fear experienced by survivors and caregivers concerns physical problems and performance. Glass (1990, p. 17) suggests that "there may be mechanical problems due to paralysis or spasticity, but, in general, there are ways to compensate for anatomical problems. The partners need to be educated. Also, there may be a need for sexual adjustments." I have found that helping caregivers understand their partner's needs, and educating them in the literature about sex after strokes, has helped them be more knowledgeable about the risks they may take in being sexually active again.

One married couple I worked with had been married for over thirty-five years, though they had often been separated for three to six months at a time due to the survivor's work schedule. As a result of this schedule, they had a relatively inactive and sporadic sex life throughout their marriage. But after his stroke, the husband became quite demanding sexually with his wife. The caregiver (wife) had difficulty complying with his demands. She was fearful that he might have another stroke and didn't like being submissive to her husband. She stated that sex was never a pleasurable experience for her but that she was committed to her husband and their marriage. After making a conscious decision to comply with her husband's demands, she stated that they did have several sexual encounters and she found she was able to experience pleasure and intimacy. She could now participate in the caring sex that she had not been able to experience before his stroke. Her husband apparently felt the need to have some control over his body and feel adequate sexually. She was able to consciously release her fears in order to satisfy her husband's needs for intimacy. I witnessed a beautiful expression of unconditional love given to this survivor by his wife.

Forgiveness

As a group leader and caregiver myself, I find forgiveness to be an essential element in bringing about peace, harmony, and healing. I sometimes suggest a self-forgiveness meditation to members of the stroke support group. Caregivers are often interested in learning about this concept. I play soft background music and ask the group members to close their eyes and do some deep breathing to relax. I then proceed to ask them to reflect on the quality of forgiveness. I focus the reflection on forgiving another person and end by encouraging them to focus on forgiving themselves. This exercise is described in Stephen Levine's *Who Dies?* (1982). It is also an effective way for the caregivers to forgive themselves for what has happened to them and their survivors. Most survivors are angry at themselves for possibly bringing on their stroke. The caregivers feel guilty about not being aware of what was going on with their survivor. It is often difficult for them to forgive themselves, too. When they are asked to forgive themselves, they release the pain they feel and open their hearts to understanding forgiveness and peace.

Some couples talk about forgiveness and releasing old issues. Some caregivers have to forgive their survivors and allow healing to occur for both of them. David and Samantha had been married forty-five years. They talked about their relationship before the stroke. There were some old wounds that the wife (caregiver) was not able to forgive. They discussed both of their needs. She had cared for him for two years and was resentful. She needed more space and privacy. He acknowledged his mistakes and wanted forgiveness. She was working on the process of forgiving, since this was the first time they had discussed these wounds from the past. We talked about living in the present and their commitment to each other as a married couple. Could she live with the hurt and resentment or could she release these feelings? This couple had a spiritual connection with each other. We discussed letting go and letting God heal them both. David cried through most of our session, and Samantha was able to comfort him and show that she could be loving and caring toward him. I received a Christmas card stating that she was moving toward a healing with her husband and progressing toward intimacy again with him.

Successes and Failures

When Bud first came into the support group, he was depressed, frustrated, and aphasic (unable to speak clearly). His children were fighting over who would care for him. He was a professional who constantly used his mind, yet now he could not release his thoughts. He continued therapy and received medication for depression. He progressed steadily with his recovery and hoped eventually to secure his driver's license. His first goal was to ride his bike to the support group. After accomplishing this goal, he was also able to express himself more and learned to write things down that he could not say. Bud began to encourage other group members, and in doing so, he encouraged himself. I was in awe of his many accomplishments and his caring attitude toward others. Soon he was able to ride the bus to the group meetings. He determined which bus route to take and began to take the bus every week.

Bud encouraged the other group members to do volunteer work—

he was himself working with handicapped children. The volunteer work helped Bud with his own self-esteem and contributed to his healing. He could speak in short phrases and used gestures to communicate at this time. His language skills had improved, and he was soon able to increase his reading skills. This remarkable man suggested a group presentation where someone could demonstrate the use of a computer for survivors with aphasia. Bud is a good example of someone who had the determination to handle this situation and come out as a person who is now experiencing a changed but fulfilling life. He would often let me know when different techniques used in group would be positive and uplifting to him.

Genevieve offers another wonderful success story. Her family wanted her to move closer to her daughter and grandchild. Prior to moving, she suffered the loss of one of her daughters as well as her husband. She had hoped the move would help her get over these losses. She had lived in the local community for about six weeks when her stroke occurred. She had loved life and enjoyed traveling but was now unable to do many of the things she enjoyed and was depressed at the time I first saw her. Genevieve joined the support group and was able to express her feelings of loss. Her family planned to go away for Christmas and wanted her to join them. However, she was afraid of flying and anxious about who would help her on and off the plane—even though the airlines do go out of their way to help disabled people.

Genevieve made the trip, visited her family, and shared her experiences with the group. She has now traveled at least three times, including going to a fiftieth wedding anniversary within her family. She is trying to resume her hobby of painting. She also attended a bereavement group and got support for her many losses. She is determined to reinvest in life and have a high-quality life. I often cry with her in our group sessions, as she shares her joy in being fully alive again.

Edith's rehabilitation was not very successful. She was a stroke survivor who had fallen in her home and was found two days later by a neighbor who went to check on her. The neighbor called 911 and Edith went to the hospital, where they determined that she had suffered a stroke. Her daughter lived out of town and was unable to care for her.

Edith's cousin was called on to help with her care. Edith thought her cousin was taking advantage of her. The cousin was willing to help out but wanted her own space. Edith needed help taking her medication and was experiencing speech problems and dementia. She became more and more isolated, staying in her room all day and only coming out to eat meals. Because of the lack of communication between the cousin and Edith, her daughter had to make other arrangements for her. Edith was placed in a nursing facility and suffered a tremendous loss. She was in her eighties and had lived in her own home for fifty years with her dogs and cats. It broke my heart to witness this loss for Edith. If the daughter had been willing to secure another type of caregiver for her, she could have stayed in her own home and experienced the security and quality of life she deserved.

I was angry and sad about the outcome of Edith's situation. I realized that the daughter had limitations and had to make a difficult decision. I get highly frustrated and annoyed thinking about these helpless and sometimes hopeless situations. I then realize that I have limitations, too. I have had to realize that other people are trying to do the best they can and accept that. It does not make it any easier, it's just reality. It's hard when you don't have control over the outcome. Even poor Edith didn't have control of her own destiny, and I have no control of her destiny either. What I can do as a social worker is to help survivors and their families look at options and recommendations for care and support them through the grieving process.

Challenges, Rewards, and Miracles

The most challenging part of my job is not taking the problems and feelings of the survivors and their families home with me. I am personally learning how to release these stressful feelings to a higher power or God, by practicing meditation, listening to relaxation music, and empowering myself spiritually. This is difficult to do. I am learning that I am doing the best I can under the circumstances and am learning how to be assertive and self-caring. Caregivers must realize that they have to take care of themselves, too. That is the biggest challenge to me.

The most difficult part of my job is working with survivors who are depressed or who could be suicidal and have no support system. Sometimes a survivor who has been relying on a spouse for several years will lose their partner through death or illness. I am concerned about what will happen to the survivor now. Who will take care of him or her? Some survivors become depressed because they don't have good coping skills or have lost those skills due to the limitations imposed by their stroke. Some survivors choose to leave the support group because it is too painful to experience the feeling of loss. The survivors who have a good support system, even if they can't speak, seem to do okay in the group and in the community, because they have the support and respect from their family and friends. The survivors with little or no support are likely to experience many difficulties in confronting their limitations and often become isolated and withdrawn from others. I have also seen cases of neglect where the survivor chose not to press charges against their alleged abusers and refused help. I worry about these survivors, but I am learning that I cannot control or change some situations.

Cases where survivors choose to stay in situations that are not positive for them make me sad and very angry. I am learning, however, that for my own self-care I can and must release these frustrations. I do this by discussing difficult cases with my husband, who is my best friend and a caring listener. I never use names or disclose confidential information about cases, but I do share my concerns and frustrations about these survivors. I also discuss these cases with my supervisor and other colleagues, who encourage me and give me feedback and a shoulder to cry on. It is absolutely necessary to have someone to listen to me, give me a sense of self-esteem, and help me realize that I am doing the best I can with these survivors.

Let me tell you about a survivor who both challenged and rewarded me. Jim was a retired mechanic. He attended group meetings for a few months after his rehab experience. He was very caring but was, as he would say, a "macho" man. Jim was deeply concerned about his wife and family. He touched many members of the group, and I was quite fond of him. There was a videotape explaining strokes that was used

during the group. Jim wanted to check out the video in order to explain his stroke more fully to his eight-year-old grandson. He was close
to his grandson and wanted him to understand what had happened to
him. The video did help to describe the limitations Jim was experiencing. During one meeting, he felt a tightness in his chest. Since he had
suffered a previous heart attack, he decided to leave the support group
early and drive himself to the hospital. He had, indeed, suffered another
heart attack. I visited him in the hospital, and he shared with me that
he was not afraid to die. He had made peace with God and with his
family. He had a priest come and give him the last sacraments, and
he felt good about his life. He was able to go home but did not return
to the support group.

A few months later, Jim suffered a massive heart attack. His wife
rushed him to the hospital, but he went into a coma and died the following day. His wife asked me to attend a memorial service at the hospital. I called the therapists at the rehab center who had worked with
Jim, and we all gathered at the chapel in the hospital. During the service, the chaplain read some of Jim's favorite poems. One of the poems
was one I had given to Jim. This was a shock to me. I had no idea that
this particular poem meant so much to him and had such an impact
in his life. The poem spoke about going beyond yourself, about healing
and recovery. It spoke about reinvesting in life and living one day at
a time. It was something that Jim really took to heart.

I cried during the service. I felt a connection to this stroke survivor. He had lived a full and good life, and he had learned to live
with his limitations. He golfed with one hand, drove his car, and helped
his wife with the vacuuming and other tasks. He touched people deeply
by his example and motivation to enjoy life. I found I had touched Jim,
too. I never realized what an influence I'd had on some survivors, the
little things that may have made a difference, a hug, words of encouragement, or even poems I'd handed out. I felt angry, sad, happy, and finally
peaceful knowing Jim was now at peace.

Growth and change are part of the process of life. After people have
experienced a stroke, they are forced to change and grow—which is
stressful. Sometimes it is a painful struggle. Survivors who have never

exercised must exercise daily to help maintain muscle tone and joint movement. They learn to eat differently, sometimes with another hand. Food tastes different, so they have a challenge in merely engaging in the daily activity of eating. Some survivors find it difficult to swallow and are embarrassed about drooling. Everything has changed for them—the way they walk, hold objects, write their name, and talk. This process of change can be overwhelming and devastating. The losses are great. Stroke survivors and caregivers are constantly fighting to improve while they are also grieving their losses.

Learning to cope with the grief, the loss, the limitations, doing things differently, and accepting help can cause survivors to deny what has happened and to avoid looking at who they are or where they are going in life. It's tough. Sometimes survivors come back to me and say, "I've tried doing that task; it didn't feel good but I did it anyway and it worked. I remember when we talked about releasing my old negative feelings and changing those into positive feelings. It helped to change my behavior." Some survivors use relaxation tapes to change, and others use daily meditation and prayer. Whatever works for a survivor is a blessing if it brings about a positive change. When survivors get in touch with their inner strength, it helps them begin the painful growth associated with surviving a stroke and recapturing their life. I have witnessed many survivors who now have a good and productive quality of life. They have learned to cope because they love life and want good things to happen, both to them and to their loved ones.

I conclude this chapter about healing and forgiveness with an Indian word that I heard at a conference on grief and loss. This word has helped me better understand the feelings of honor and praise I have for stroke survivors and their families. The word is *namaste*. According to Ken Moses, who discussed this in a workshop presented in San Francisco in 1993, the English translation of this word is as follows: "I honor the place in you in which the universe dwells. I honor the place in you which is of love, of truth, of light, and of peace. When you are in that place in you, and I am in that place in me, we are one." To all stroke survivors and caregivers, past and future, I gently offer with great appreciation and respect, *Namaste*.

Epilogue

Since this book was written, Barbara Kobylinski has accepted the challenge of using her gifts in other areas of the medical/healing profession. She is currently working as a medical social worker in an acute hospital setting. She works with patients experiencing short-term, progressive, and terminal illness as well as giving support to their families. She continues to encourage these patients to empower themselves in their healing and recovery process.

Bill Bergquist has also moved on to the exploration of other types of intrusive life events—ranging from the confrontation of men and women in Eastern Europe with the prospects of increased freedom and responsibility to the adjustment of adults to catastrophic life events. In each case, he goes back to the extraordinary stories that he has heard and read about stroke survivors and caregivers making new sense of their shattered lives and literally reconstructing their world of language, movement, emotions, and interpersonal relationships. Rod McLean and Barabara Kobylinski have both served as exceptional guides in leading Bill—as someone from outside the field—to a greater appreciation of the exceptional courage and commitment exhibited by the stroke survivors and caregivers featured in this book.

In our study of stroke survivors and caregivers, we focused primarily on the period between the occurrence of a stroke and the transition back home following rehabilitation from the stroke. This is a uniquely challenging and sometimes rewarding period in the lives of stroke survivors and caregivers. Life, of course, moves on after a stroke survivor returns home. The survivor and caregiver face new challenges as they reestablish their individual lives as well as their lives together.

The majority of the stroke survivors and caregivers included in this book are still leading productive and fulfilling—but changed—lives. Most continue to attend stroke survivor groups. A few survivors have dropped out of the groups but are active in their community as volunteer workers—assisting other, more recent stroke survivors. A few survivors and caregivers keep in touch just to inform Barbara or Rod that they are continuing to grow, change, and accept their quality of life after the stroke. Several of the people we interviewed have died, either from another stroke or from other causes.

For Rod, the acceptance of his stroke experience has taken many different forms: more education, advocacy, teaching, and consulting—and the coauthoring of this book. Due to his "brain attack" and because of having been a stroke survivor for several years, Rod has passed many milestones. There are some wonderful memories, as he watched actual miracles happening, and all the while his soul grew stronger as he moved closer to what he wanted. At the same time, he has many memories of incidents that were ridiculous, emotionally traumatic, absurd, and against his principles. He often felt anger, as he was constantly being misunderstood, discriminated against, and rejected by individuals, groups, and entire systems.

Rod recalls that on being released from the hospital after a long regimen of intensive therapies, he devised his own program of exercises and enrolled in some bonehead college English courses. Still operating in a survival mode, he decided to continue with college. The intensity of the classes and their requirements were compounded by stroke-caused deficits: short-term memory loss and difficulties in expressing anything. The main reasons for taking the classes were to continue his efforts to improve his communication skills, to increase his cognitive abilities, to figure out what he was going to do with the rest of his life, and even to get some good grades. For quite a while, he wanted desperately not to be disabled. He wanted to be "normal." So, in a way, he was fighting to get away from the person that he had become and the painful role he now occupied.

Over time, he realized that he would strongly enjoy teaching and working with children, especially those who are challenged. He persisted in his efforts to acquire the academic credentials needed to teach in the field of special education. It was tough studying for the many required courses. It took him six years—rather than the usual four—to earn a bachelor's degree. He was so happy and proud to have accomplished the task that virtually everyone said he couldn't accomplish. But he wasn't satisfied. He felt that there were still more mountains to climb. To reach an even more difficult summit, it took him another six years to obtain a master's degree in psychology.

After a while, he taught and counseled disabled children and adults of all sizes, shapes, ages, cognitive levels, physical abilities, and attitudes. It was all very satisfying. He believes he helped many of them, and, at a deep level, he knows that every one of them taught him exactly what he was supposed to learn.

He realized that he needed to share with many other people his miracle of living through a massive stroke. He began by talking about his experiences with children in a second-grade classroom. It was so scary! He had to expose his weaknesses. That meant baring the parts of him that he was so embarrassed about—why he walks oddly with a limp, why he has so much difficulty speaking, how he omits words or doesn't say the words correctly. He thought thirty seven-year-olds were going to massacre his soul. But the kids were great! They all gave him hugs and thanks! It felt right! As he was leaving the school, he recognized that the burden of embarrassment he had carried with him since his stroke had lifted. It was replaced by a sense of pride, as he began to represent disabled people in his work. He realized that this point in time signaled a wonderful new beginning. It became easier to believe in himself. Knowing that he would be able to give so much more, a feeling of warmth and wellness came over him!

A decade and thousands of presentations later, he finally felt secure enough to present himself to his stroke survivor peers. To him, it was frightening in that he was himself in each and every one of them. He saw himself at all stages of rehabilitation. He reexperienced the pain, anguish, and fear of being in a new and crazy world. He saw all of his stroke experiences in their eyes and felt their souls touch his. He gave them his heart. They acknowledged and accepted who and where he was. They showed him that they had been there together. They gave him the motivation to strongly advocate for all survivors. These people provided him with the drive he needed to finally be part of this book.

We hope that this will be just the beginning, as the door opens for millions of stroke survivors and enables them to find the empowerment and independence—and above all, the fulfilling lives—they so richly deserve.

The Authors

William H. Bergquist is president of the Professional School of Psychology, a graduate school that primarily serves mature, accomplished adults, with campuses in San Francisco and Sacramento, California. He received his B.A. degree (1962) from Occidental College, Los Angeles, in psychology and his M.A. degree (1965) and Ph.D. degree (1969) from the University of Oregon, also in psychology. He has written or coauthored more than twenty books on adult development, organizational cultures, the experience of freedom in Eastern Europe, psychological adaptation to strokes, and the nature of our emerging postmodern era. Bergquist has served as a consultant to more than 300 corporations, human service agencies, collegiate institutions, and churches throughout the United States, Canada, Eastern Europe, and Asia. He lives with his wife, Kathleen, on the Mendocino coast in Northern California and is a proud father of two and grandfather of two.

Rod McLean is a "brain attack" survivor who suffered a severe aneurysm a quarter of a century ago at age twenty, which left him completely paralyzed on one side and unable to communicate. After years of arduous rehabilitation, he obtained his B.A. degree (1974) from Evergreen State College, Olympia, in special education and his M.A. degree (1980) from Antioch University/West, Seattle, in psychology, and is now working on his Psy.D. at the Professional School of Psychology. McLean has devoted himself to assisting other challenged individuals striving to

reenter the mainstream of life. His national ABLEforce business, founded
in 1979 in San Rafael, California, was initially dedicated to raising disability awareness among students and adults, laypeople and professionals,
caregivers and survivors. His consulting service has expanded to provide
"Americans with Disabilities Act" training for corporations, government
entities, and nonprofit institutions. McLean has published a disability
awareness manual, *Challenges for Children,* and writes "Sharing from a
Survivor," a bimonthly newsletter column that addresses questions asked
by those affected by a stroke, whether they be survivors, health workers, or loved ones.

Barbara A. Kobylinski is a social worker at Mercy San Juan/Mercy
American River Hospitals in Sacramento, California. She received both
her B.A. (1989) and M.S.W. (1990) degrees from Florida State University, Tallahassee, in social work. She has worked with chemically dependent adolescents at a residential treatment center in Tallahassee
and for Foster Care and Adoption Services, a division of the Florida
Department of Health and Rehabilitation Services. She completed a
master's degree internship at the Florida State University Student Counseling Center. As a social worker at the Mercy Regional Center for
Rehabilitation, she counseled stroke survivors and their families. She
facilitated stroke and caregiver groups and led a stroke therapy group.
She lives with her husband Gerry and her daughter Stacie and son Tony
in Sacramento.

The Research Team

Sally Arnold

Constance J. Arburua

Laura M. Castro

Rosalind J. Ewell

Jeffrey P. Hardesty

Carrie A. Harper

Harold H. Johnson

F. Jeanne Johnson

Sara Joslyn

Barbara Lancaster

Soonja Choi Lee

Elaine Economo Mangan

Robert B. McVaugh

Thomas Moon

Judy J. Morris

Pamela Morrison

Darrell Parent

Robert J. Patla

Tony Paulson

Linda J. Sanchez

Roya Sakhai

Marie Scannell

Deborah K. Schmidt

Gus Shelton

Barbara Singleton

Marcy Stites

Lorain Tremayne-Cummings

Linda K. Tucker

Carmen Valdez

Donald Wallach

Kathleen Walsh

Maxine Wester Williams

Beverly Winslow

Heidi Dobrzak Wright

References

Alzheimer's Society. *Caregiver's Bill of Rights.* "Yes I Can" Workshop. Sacramento, Calif.: Alzheimer's Society, 1992.

Fromm, E. *The Art of Loving.* New York: HarperCollins, 1956.

Glass, D. "There Is Sex After Stroke." *Be Stroke Smart.* Englewood, Colo.: National Stroke Association, 1990.

Hay, L. *Ten Steps to Loving Yourself.* Compton, Calif.: Hay House, 1993.

Holmes, T., and Rahe, R. "The Social Readjustment Rating Scale." *Journal of Psychosomatic Research,* 1967, *11,* 213–218.

Kübler-Ross, E. *On Death and Dying.* New York: Macmillan, 1969.

Levine, S. *Who Dies?* New York: Anchor Press/Doubleday, 1982.

National Stroke Association. *The Road Ahead: A Stroke Recovery Guide.* Englewood, Colo.: National Stroke Association, 1986.

Rahe, R., McKean, J., and Arthur, R. "A Longitudinal Study of Life-Change and Illness Patterns." *Journal of Psychosomatic Research,* 1967, *11,* 213–218

Schmall, V., and Stiehl, R. *Coping with Caregiving: How to Manage Stress When Caring for Elderly Relatives.* Corvallis, Oreg.: Pacific Northwest Extension, Oregon State University, 1989.

Shimberg, E. *Strokes: What Families Should Know*. New York: Random House, 1990.

Siegel, B. *Meditations for Peace of Mind/Healing Images, Affirmations/ A Positive New You Affirmations*. Audiotapes: Rx for Living Series. New Haven, Conn.: ECap, 1990a.

Siegel, B. *Peace, Love, and Healing*. New York: HarperCollins, 1990b.

Zelman, D. "Race, Culture, Values, and Strokes." Unpublished manuscript, Berkeley, Calif., 1992.

Index